GUIDE TO HEALTHY AGING AFTER 50

What You Need To Know

Don Everett Bitle

◆ FriesenPress

Suite 300 - 990 Fort St
Victoria, BC, V8V 3K2
Canada

www.friesenpress.com

Copyright © 2017 by Don Everett Bitle
First Edition — 2017

All rights reserved.

No part of this publication may be reproduced in any form, or by any means, electronic or mechanical, including photocopying, recording, or any information browsing, storage, or retrieval system, without permission in writing from FriesenPress.

ISBN
978-1-5255-0527-0 (Hardcover)
978-1-5255-0528-7 (Paperback)
978-1-5255-0529-4 (eBook)

1. BISAC *code 001*

Distributed to the trade by The Ingram Book Company

TABLE OF CONTENTS

The Introduction
1

Chapter 1:
Make Sure You Are Healthy Enough
5

Chapter 2:
Avoiding Some Bad Habits
13

Chapter 3:
Exercise and What It Really Takes
23

Chapter 4:
We Are What We Eat
37

Chapter 5:
Focus Also on The Brain
43

Chapter 6:
Focus On What You Are Able to Do
47

References:
51

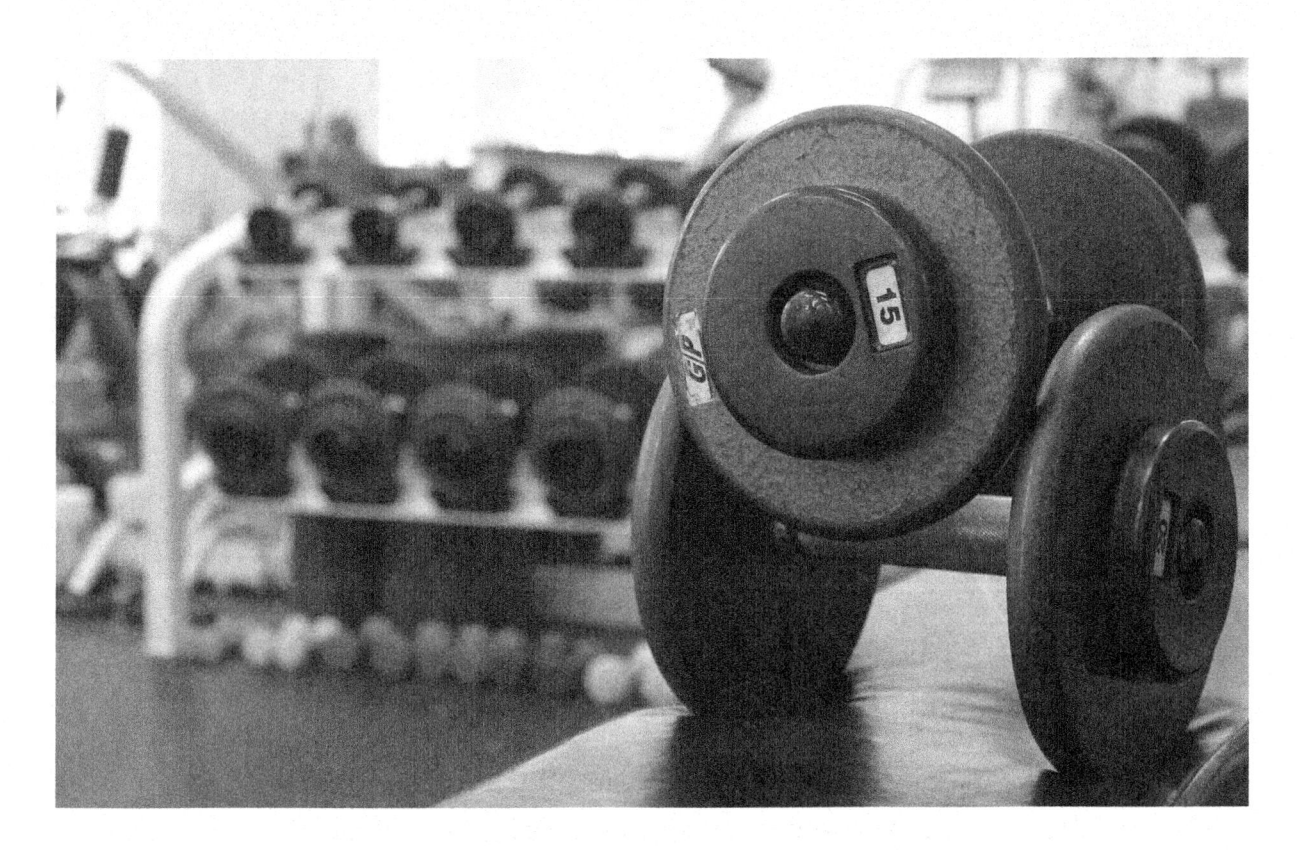

THE INTRODUCTION

I'm writing *Guide* to *Healthy Aging After 50* for all those men and women who want to be and stay healthy during their senior years. This group ranges in age from fifty to 100+ years old. I selected this fifty-year period because this is the demographic I work with every day. These are the men and women on whom I focus in my personal training and class instructions. This guide to healthy aging will specifically examine many of the issues and challenges members of this age group encounter every day.

I will explain these challenges and issues as I try to lead you to a better, healthier lifestyle. The lifestyle an individual leads can usually predict how well and how long he/she will live.

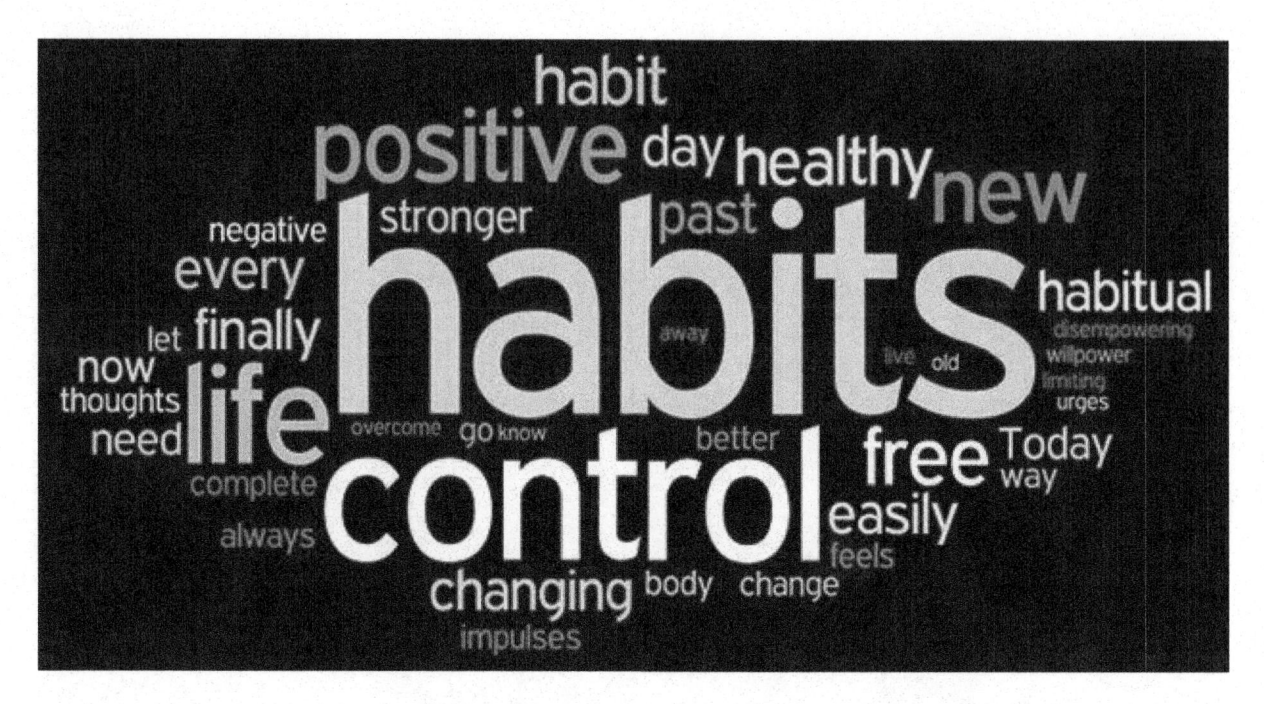

We always have reasons not to take things seriously.

The first fifty years of life are the lifestyle years. What do I mean by that?

These lifestyle years, or what can also be called the addiction or habit years, have a profound effect on preventive care, nutrition, physical activity, and other issues our demographic suffers. It's during those early years that we learn the good and bad habits that take us into the next fifty years. In those early years, we form our habits regarding healthy practices.

These early lifestyle habits may have included issues like smoking, heavy drinking, overeating, using serious street drugs, dangerous driving, and dangerous sports and exercises, all of which we usually regret after entering our fifties. Let's look at some examples:

Take the habit of eating. We all need to eat. When we are younger, we don't think too much about what we put into our mouths. We sometimes overeat and build an addiction to poor choices, such as fast, fad, unclean, and processed foods. We've all had experience with what bad eating habits do to our bodies. In our twenties, thirties, forties, and sometimes our fifties, we can eat these foods and not be affected by the consequences that hit us in our senior years. We see our weight go up, maybe an increase in our blood pressure, or issues with diseases such as chronic obstructive pulmonary disease (COPD), diabetes, heart diseases, and LDL (bad) cholesterol. And

THE INTRODUCTION

I haven't even mentioned other problems that come along such as cancers, arthritis, gout, other joint pains, etc. Now some of these issues are related to causes besides foods, but you get my point. "We are what we eat," but we can change these poor food habits, and that is one reason I've written this book. Sadly, younger generations are also seeing these problems.

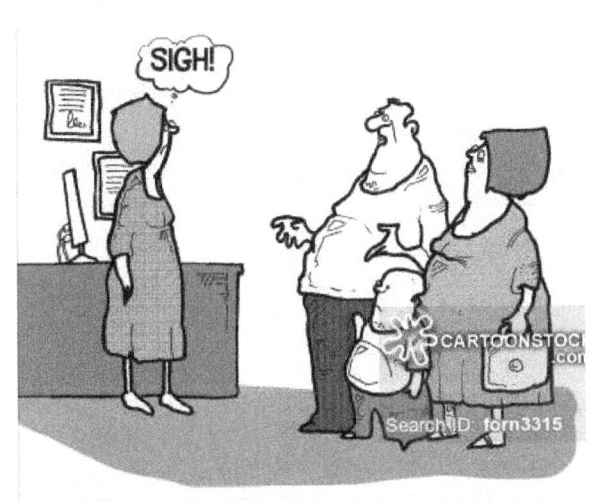

Preventive care for seniors such as health screenings, vaccinations, and written knowledge from books, magazines, etc., have given us an edge on what we can use to help us as we age. Poor nutrition affects our health. Lack of physical activity affects our health. Even the use of our time affects our health.

I'll use one more example to help us focus on changing our lifestyle. This is exercise. Physical exercise for seniors is still statistically less thought of than most groups. According to the latest statistics, Americans fifty-five years of age and over spend more than fifty percent of their leisure time watching TV, reading, and sitting in front of computers playing games, and only do small amounts of physical activities such as cleaning the house, gardening, or working. Now don't get me wrong. We do need to do these things once in a while. Cleaning and yardwork are exercise, and the sooner you start these good things, the healthier you will be in your senior years. But we can do more!

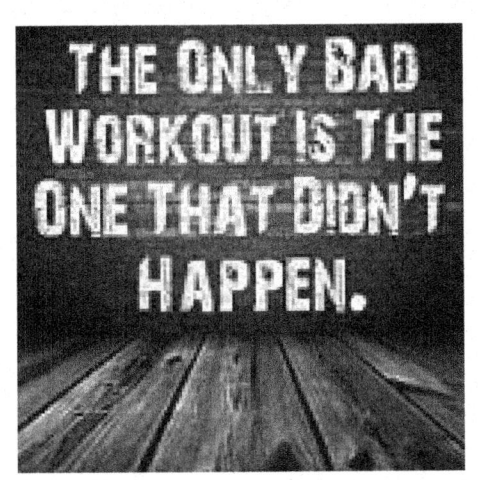

Now that we have established the reasons to embrace a healthy, active lifestyle, let's see what we need to do to keep us healthy going forward.

CHAPTER 1:
Make Sure You Are Healthy Enough

The **American College of Sports Medicine** (ACSM) suggests we should be able to exercise five days a week for at least sixty minutes a day, with appropriate recommendations for each person's risk stratification. As we get older, some of us are not quite healthy enough to dive right into a lot of exercise if we haven't been doing it for years. ALWAYS be smart about what your body can handle and use common sense when you start an exercise regime.

Perhaps you might start with just walking, or riding a bike a few miles a day. How you feel after these small steps can determine how much further you can push yourself. Anything to get you into a pattern of exercise will encourage you to do more.

These risk stratifications categories—or what we call *risk factors*—are based on strong recommendations designed to help each individual reach their fitness levels, as determined by their cardiorespiratory endurance, muscle strength, balance, agility, and flexibility.

All personal trainers, group exercise instructors, as well as doctors, physical therapists, etc., should know what their client stratification category is.

The ACSM Risk Stratification Categories are:

1. **Low risk:** Men and women who have zero or one risk factor and no symptoms. These symptoms would be things like heart problems, obesity, cardiorespiratory issues, etc. If you have no risk, then go all out on your exercise and work four or five days a week for sixty minutes or more.

2. **Moderate risk:** Men and women who have two or more risk factors and no symptoms. Let's say you have a weight problem and you want to lose fifteen

or twenty pounds, because your blood pressure is slightly elevated. This would be a moderate risk factor that could be corrected by weight loss, diet, and exercise. Working out with weights and some cardio for sixty minutes, two to three days a week, could put you back into the low-risk class, and that is your goal.

3. **High risk:** Individuals who have known cardiovascular, pulmonary, or metabolic disease; or one or more signs and symptoms of cardiovascular, pulmonary, or metabolic disease. This group must exercise caution. Just having them walk or move will help. The more exercise they do (two or three days at thirty to forty-five minutes) can really change this risk stratification.

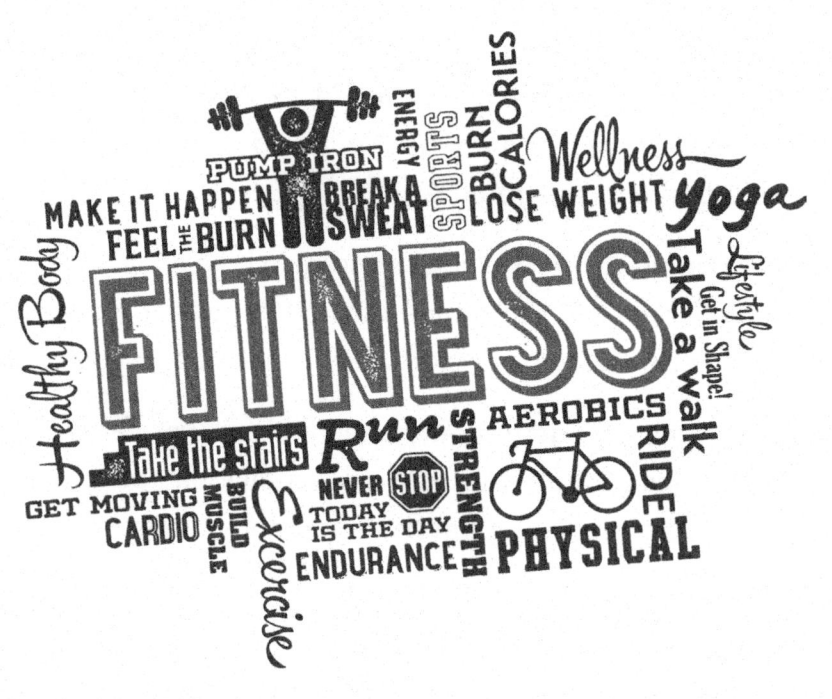

Even the activities we perform on a daily basis—such as walking, sitting, standing, stair-climbing, reaching, and dressing—are relevant to our well-being and quality of life. Programs designed for these risk categories will help all who consult a health professional at a gym. I highly recommend conducting some form of health screening to identify health risks in relationship to exercise. The Physical Activity Readiness Questionnaire (PAR-Q) or some other orientation form is needed for your safety and the gym you go to. These evaluations help protect the client/participant from unnecessary harm, and are important for protecting you (or the club/facility) from a legal and insurance perspective. **Always check with your doctor before starting an exercise program.**

CHAPTER 1: MAKE SURE YOU ARE HEALTHY ENOUGH

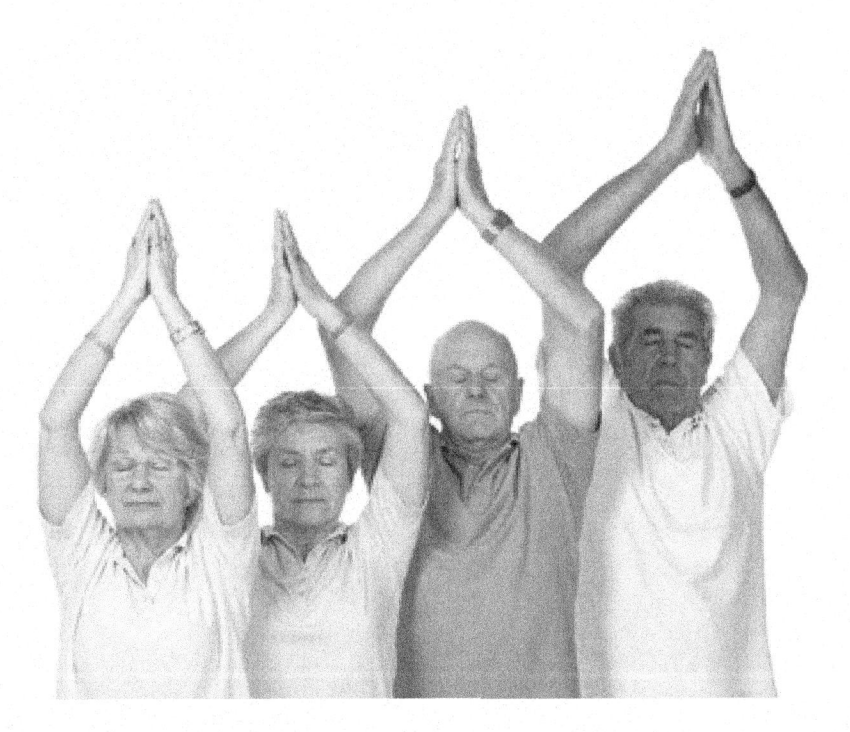

Having an understanding of the varying fitness levels among older adults can also help in choosing the right program for skill-related exercises. Cardiovascular (heart), strength, flexibility, and balance training are very important. The big problem is: if we do an exercise wrong and/or we hurt ourselves, what will that do to us?

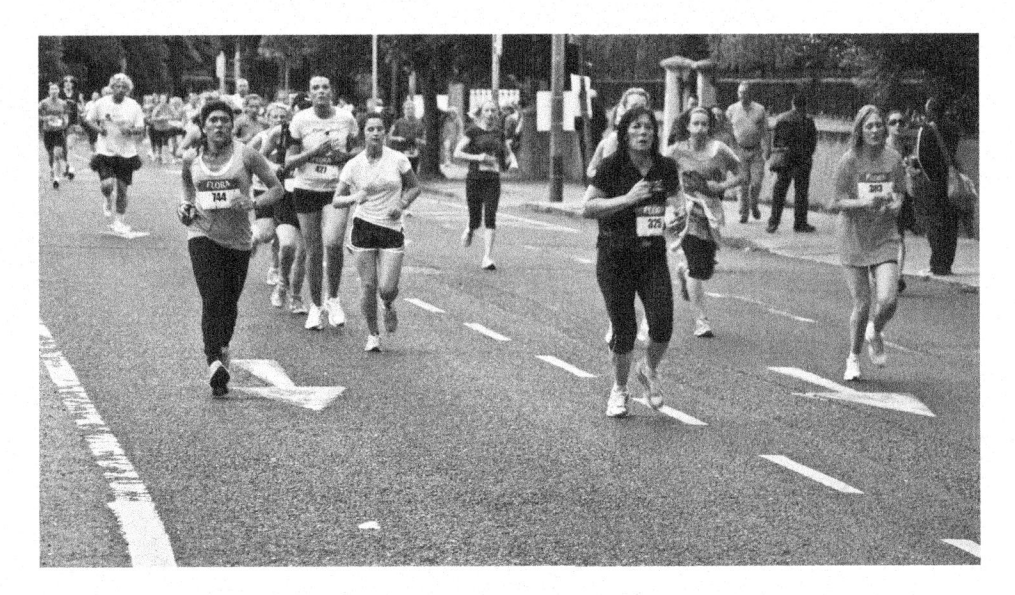

In 2014, a National Public Health Week Survey found that seventy-eight percent of Americans fifty-five years of age and older understand that exercise is important in determining how healthy they will be as they age, but the fear of getting injured was a big reason for not participating in any physical activity. Other negative factors included: advanced age, low income, lack of time, low motivation, a perception that a great effort is needed to exercise, rural residency, being overweight or obese, being physically or mentally disabled, and even the perception of what health is. Negative attitudes toward physical activity and exercise and lack of support or encouragement by others (including people you trust, like healthcare professionals, family members, and friends) add to these, as well.

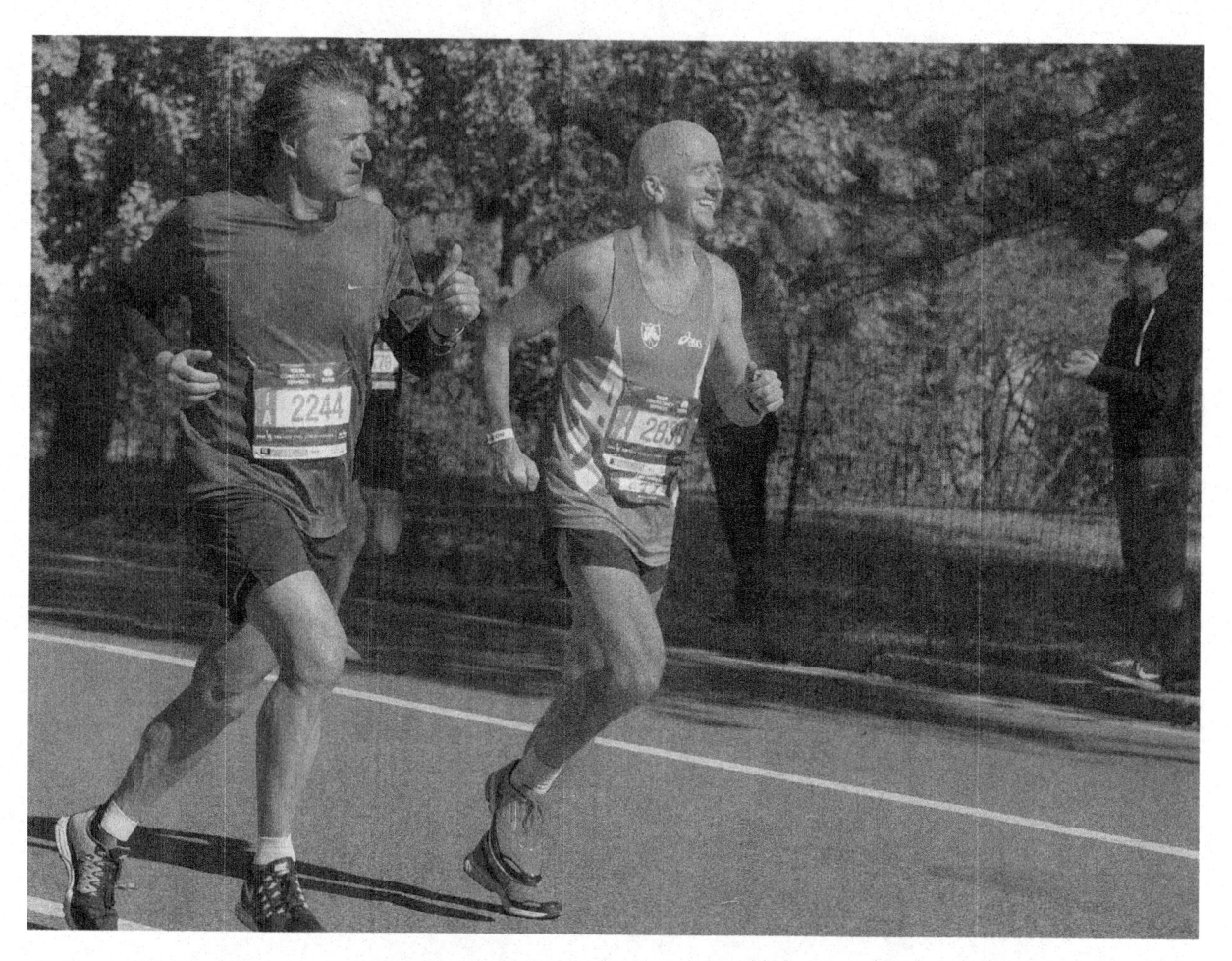

On another note, especially for the women reading this book, if workouts aren't your thing, or a gym is not available, just walking, biking, or doing the normal things in life that you do best, are better than nothing. Any movement for thirty to sixty minutes a day can benefit you tremendously.

VARY YOUR WORKOUTS

From my own experience, it is important to switch our workouts often to prevent injuries. Don't do the same thing day after day. Take running, for example. I grew up

CHAPTER 1: MAKE SURE YOU ARE HEALTHY ENOUGH

in Eugene, Oregon, and have lived in this beautiful city for over fifty years. This is the track-town city for all of the United States. I used to run all the time, but when I was in my thirties, I added weightlifting to my training. Some of my friends and co-runners just kept running, and now, as they have gotten older, have serious knee (ACL, PCL) and hip problems. Some of them suffered so badly that they are not able to exercise anymore.

I don't have any of those problems because I changed my running habits. I set up certain helpful goals for myself that I will share with you in this book. Briefly, I will say that I include stretches, leg workouts with weights, yoga, dancing, and bicycling in this regime. This has helped my bones, muscles, and tendons, and made me stronger. Weightlifting gave my legs support near the knees and hips, and helped with my gait. Weightlifting for my upper body has given me strength in my shoulders, back, chest, and arms. Yoga has taught me to stretch and has made my core stronger. Dancing and bicycling helped me with balance and sudden leg movements. If you don't believe that changing up your workouts, cross-training, and other things will help you, then do it for a while, and see for yourself. I found that it really helped me, especially with my balance.

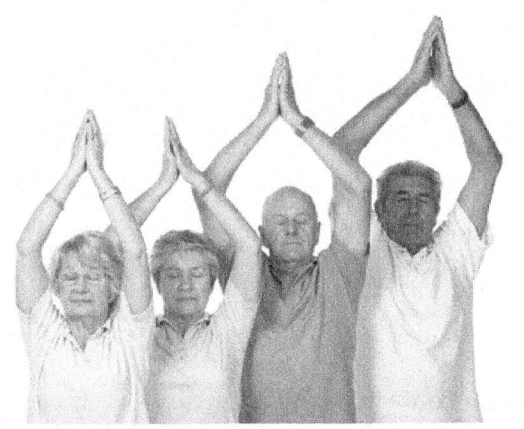

Balance issues are a big problem for aging adults. What causes these balance issues as we age?

As we grow older, most of us spend less and less time standing, reaching, and moving, and more and more time sitting. This sedentary life choice robs us of the sense and stimulation we need to keep us upright and moving.

How is your balance?

Balance is a skill that gets better with practice and worse with disuse, similar to riding a bicycle, cooking that favorite dish, or mastering a crossword puzzle. When you stop using this skill by not doing these things on a regular basis, you start having balance issues. You also forget how to ride that bike, you don't remember what goes in that favorite dish, and you have trouble working on that crossword.

To counteract this process of decline, you need to be doing balance exercises that challenge your sense of balance on a regular basis. The leg muscles are incredibly important in terms of independence and quality of life. They are also important in balance, because they are the muscles that actually move your legs, ankles, and feet.

After age fifty, according to science, we lose about one percent of our leg strength per year. That can add up after a few decades. This, and our sedentary life choices, really contribute to balance issues as we grow older.

Practice balance exercises every day. As an example of a balance exercise, try this: Stand next to something sturdy like a kitchen or bathroom sink. Put one foot in front of the other (touch heel to tip of toes), with one hand holding onto the countertop for support. As you begin to feel comfortable in this position, slowly let go of the counter and hold for a few seconds. As you build this skill, try to balance in this position for thirty seconds. Turn around and do the same position with the other foot in front. Do this with your eyes open until you feel confident enough to try it with your eyes closed.

Because the legs are also important for better balance, try standing in front of a sturdy chair, and slowly squat down to the chair ten times. If you need to hold onto something, have another sturdy chair in front . Work up to more reps (fifteen to twenty times).

Another good exercise is to sit comfortably in a chair, bring one leg out and lift the foot off the floor. Begin to move the ankle in a circle one way and then the other (about ten times in each direction). Reverse this exercise with the other foot. This helps strengthen the ankles. Also, walk as much as you can during the day, as this also builds up your leg strength. Taking dance and stretching classes, like tai chi or yoga (because these classes work the legs, ankles, and feet even better than walking) can also improve your balance and reduce your risk of falling. When doing these things regularly, you can actually slow or reverse the balance problem.

CHAPTER 1: MAKE SURE YOU ARE HEALTHY ENOUGH

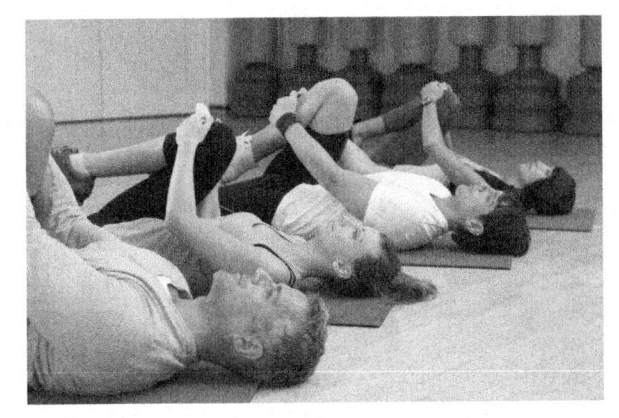

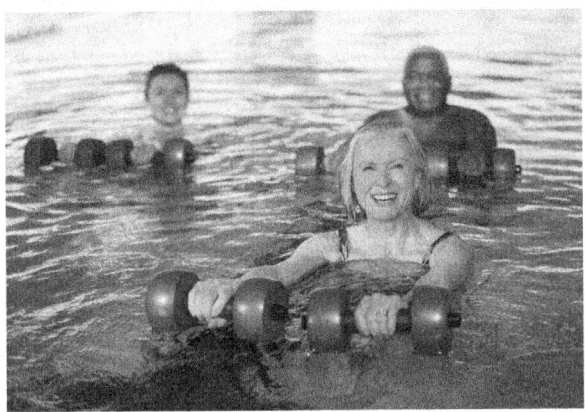

As an aerobic instructor for active seniors for the last ten years, I constantly change my workouts. I have my students and clients use weights for upper and lower body parts. I have them do dance movements that help them with their balance. I include stretches for flexibility before and after workouts. **AND I NEVER** tell them to do something that may harm their bodies. If it will hurt me, then it will hurt them, and they are more precious than anything.

So, as I continue to remind the reader, it is during the first fifty years that we form our lifestyle habits, and very few men and women choose healthy habits that will benefit them after fifty. Now that we have made it into fifties, sixties, seventies, eighties, nineties, and on into the hundreds, I'm here to tell you what is possible. Our bodies are able to heal from bad habits. They are able to change. It doesn't take a long time. You can see changes in weeks.

These are just some examples that I will refer to again as we move forward.

SET GOALS

You must follow some rules. You must want to change. You must set goals and take control of everything that failed you in the past. You must want to start, and to be consistent, persistent, and honest about your goals. Otherwise, you will not have the health you want.

The real goal and current wave for senior exercisers is that of FUNCTIONAL FITNESS. Functional fitness helps to reduce the risk of many major diseases and illnesses. It refers to a level of strength, endurance, cardiovascular efficiency, joint flexibility, and balance that enable us to carry out the activities of daily living (ADLs) effectively.

CHAPTER 2:
Avoiding Some Bad Habits

SMOKING: Do you smoke cigarettes, cigars or pipes; chew tobacco; or use e-cigarettes? It's not hard to start them—but it is to quit. My parents both smoked cigarettes because it was the socially acceptable thing to do. So did some of my brothers. My dad was able to quit cigarettes, but not his pipe or his chew. My mom and one of my brothers could not quit, and I remember when I tried it myself as a teenager. It's going to be hard to quit smoking now that we can smoke marijuana. Soon, it will be accepted by every state. So the times haven't changed, just the habit. Do you inhale smoke? Don't! Tobacco and marijuana contain chemical carcinogens, toxins, and other cancer-causing agents when you smoke them.

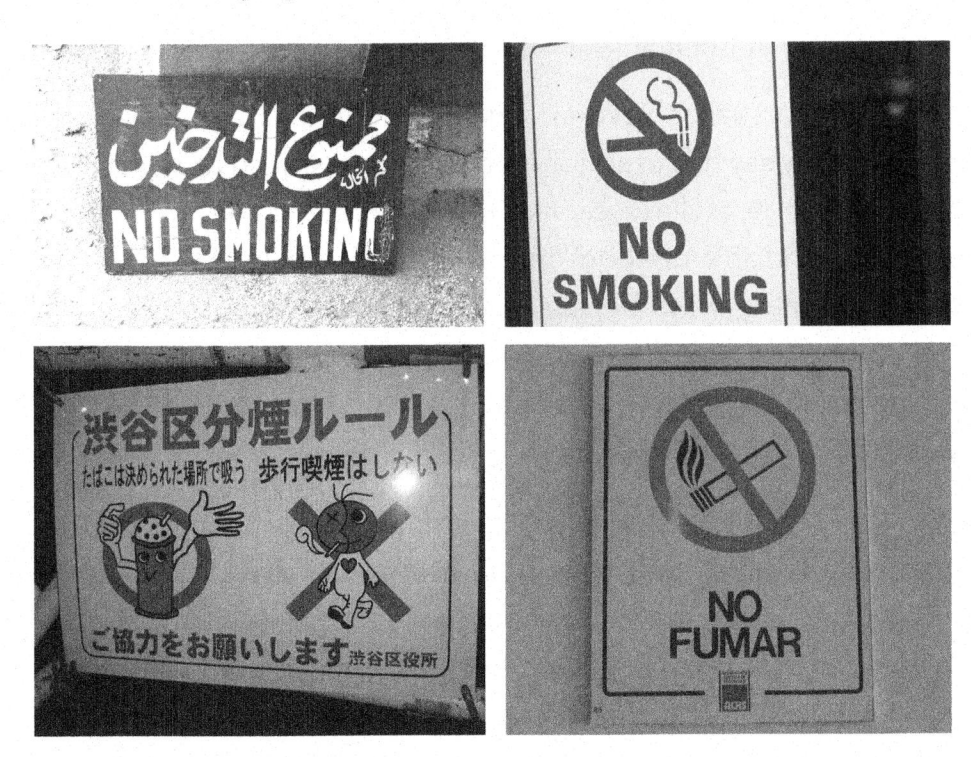

Smoking is bad in any language

Over 500,000 people in the United States will come down with smoking-related health issues every year. Out of those, more than a third will not recover and will die before their time. Those of us in the health industry see what it can do to our bodies. When I do physical orientations, I will know that a person smokes even before they tell me. Besides how bad they smell to non-smokers, they open their mouth to show their yellow teeth and tongue. And don't forget those eyes and how cloudy they are. The skin is usually lined and sagging. Do you want to look like this? Smoking causes aging.

You have probably seen the TV ads or the pictures of people who talk through a hole in their throat tell us about what smoking has done to them. So sad. Why would you want to continue to smoke when you see what it does to others? It's a bad habit, folks, and you need to quit. Putting smoke in your lungs causes a lot of diseases. It dries up the inside of the body faster than anything. Did you know that we are nearly seventy-five percent water? When you dry the body, you suffer. Do you complain about your throat, voice, chest, and skin? Then you need to stop smoking. Also, it has been noted that a growing number of companies will not hire smokers, saying they raise health-insurance costs and miss work more often than non-smokers. The smoking rate is about twenty percent among all adults, except those sixty-five and older. They're half as likely to light up. You're on the right road to good health if you quit, or never started in the first place.

Another note on marijuana. Several states, including Oregon, have passed laws making it legal. Many say it is used for medical reasons, such as relieving pain associated with a wide range of illnesses, like AIDS and some cancers. Most people will smoke marijuana, and this method of inhaling is no better than inhaling tobacco. This is amusing in many ways because a lack of useful clinical-trial data—through randomized, controlled, double-blind trials involving large patient populations—is the biggest hurdle facing marijuana's legitimacy. And yet we want to inhale this carcinogen because it might relieve pain.

It has been well established that if you quit smoking, you can clear up your lungs within three to six months. Bronchial respiratory volume increases, lungs clear up, and pulmonary cavities of the thorax improve—all within a short time. When you exercise, you open up these areas with fresh air, cleaning out the old residue from the smoke of tobacco, marijuana, or any other thing you smoke into your lungs. Don't smoke!

CHAPTER 2: AVOIDING SOME BAD HABITS

DRINKING: I'm not talking about a glass or two of wine, beer, coffee, tea. These drinks have been with us for thousands of years. It's the amount we consume that hurts our bodies. And it's the newer types of drinks that affect us even more, such as sugary drinks, sodas, all those energy drinks, and, of course, hard liquor. When we overindulge, our bodies suffer. It's interesting that a limited amount of wine and beer is OK, but when we consume more than what the body can handle, we overdose. It's recommended that women never drink more than two glasses of beer or wine a day, and men never drink more than three. It has been said that more than two-and-a-half alcoholic drinks a day over a ten-year period can cause memory loss in both male and female drinkers. We have enough problems remembering where we put our keys or why we've gone into a room. We really don't need to add to this problem, do we?

When we were young, if we got drunk, we could pass it over the next day with a hangover and recover pretty fast. It's not the same as we reach middle age and older. It can take days to recover from a drinking binge, and It has been proven that excessive drinking can cause our bodies to change over time. Excessive drinking takes the body into a tailspin. It depletes vitamins and proteins. It creates fat, softens muscles, and gives us liver/kidney problems and skin issues. Wow! Why would we want to do this to ourselves? Whether or not you avoid alcohol is an individual decision determined by both your personal preferences and risk of disease.

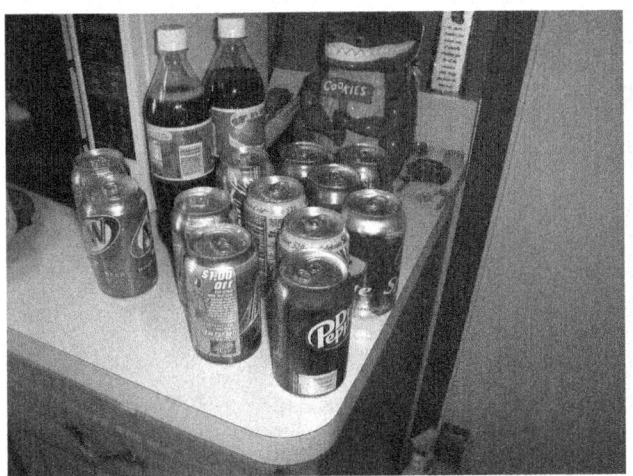

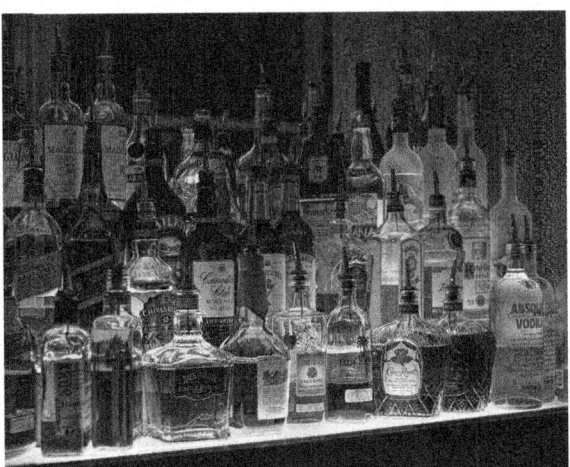

Recent studies have shown that moderate drinking can help protect the heart by raising the level of HDL "good" cholesterol and prevent blood from clotting. But your enjoyment of a glass of wine or beer can be offset if you have a personal or family history of alcoholism, breast or colon problems, etc. Consider avoiding or rarely drinking alcohol for this reason. Below are a few "standard" drinks and the amount of alcohol they contain:

12 fl oz of regular beer:
about 5% alcohol
8–9 fl oz of malt liquor
(in a 12 oz glass):
about 7% alcohol
5 fl oz of table wine:
about 12% alcohol

1.5 fl oz shot of 80-proof spirits (whiskey, gin, rum, vodka, tequila, etc.):
about 40% alcohol
The percent of "pure" alcohol, expressed here as alcohol by volume (alc/vol) varies by beverage.
(www.cheers.org.nz/standard-drinks)

A lot of sugary drinks, diet drinks, and sodas have corrosive properties that affect teeth enamel, cause weight gain, and lower the natural nutrients and supplements that are in our bodies. They are not worth it. Just drink water if you're thirsty—I do. Remember that energy drinks, soft drinks, and sodas haven't been around long and are a new temptation in our lives. More people are getting obese, diabetes, and other diseases because of them. Avoid them!

As for teas and coffee, studies have found that they should also be consumed in moderation. That said, studies have also found that regularly drinking them might reduce the risk of Type 2 diabetes by helping to regulate blood sugar, reduce some types of depression, and even lower the risk of Alzheimer's disease, colon cancer, and Parkinson's disease. Coffee also contains magnesium and potassium. Just don't overdo the caffeine. Most healthy adults can safely consume up to 300 milligrams of caffeine daily. That's about three eight-ounce cups of coffee. If you suffer from anxiety, headaches, palpitations, or tremors, you might want to reduce or eliminate these caffeine beverages to see if it helps. So it's up to your personal feelings about drinking these types of liquids. Water is still the best and cheapest source of hydration for the body.

CHAPTER 2: AVOIDING SOME BAD HABITS

"Up to 400 milligrams of **caffeine** a day appears to be safe for most healthy adults. That's roughly the amount of **caffeine** in four cups of brewed **coffee**, ten cans of cola or two "energy shot" drinks. Although **caffeine** use may be safe for adults, it's not a good idea for children."

<u>Caffeine: How much is too much? - Mayo Clinic</u>
www.mayoclinic.org/healthy-lifestyle/nutrition.../caffeine/art-20045678

Another warning about too much caffeine: the controversy around energy drinks has spread to food. You can buy caffeine-laced waffles, maple syrup, and even jelly beans and gum. If you've ever had one cup of coffee too many, you know how easy it is to overdo it. **Just be aware of everything that goes in your body.**

Another interesting note about that red wine you like to consume: Wine isn't a magical youth elixir or the fountain of youth, but it does have resveratrol from the skin of grapes which mimics the effects of calorie restriction. This is a therapy whose life-extending benefits in lab animals have been well documented. Eating a low-calorie diet that has resveratrol in it has been associated with not only a lower body mass index, but also lower blood pressure and some improved memory. The bottom line on wine then? Drink it in moderation.

DRUGS: This is not only about vitamins and supplements. With the increase in all types of health issues, doctors seem to focus on prescribed drugs of choice, with names that I can't even pronounce. And there are literally thousands of types. From NSAIDs (nonsteroidal anti-inflammatory drugs), to diabetes, obesity, and heart drugs, we have it all. We don't understand too much about them. We rely on our doctors and trust them to make us better. It's very scary when we don't know what prescription drugs do to us. Now those of us in our fifties, sixties, seventies, and eighties just blindly take them for everything from headaches to gout—"from head to toe." We use them to cover up our pain, and this can make the problems worse. Be aware of side effects. Try natural things first, such as healthful compounds called polyphenols and antioxidants, along with regular physical activity. Alternative medicines and pain-control clinics can be helpful.

There are many non-drug alternative methods to relieve pain, such as massage, acupuncture, and chiropractic and physical therapeutic remedies. Always check with a qualified doctor to see if these methods are appropriate. I use them myself and

I very seldom take any pain pills. Do what you can to educate yourself about what might be causing your pain.

Helping relieve pain safely is important, but determining which pain pills we actually need for anything from a mild headache to relieving post-surgery pain can be worrisome. Americans spend more than $2 billion a year on over-the-counter painkillers and nine times that on prescription drugs for pain. Nine times more!

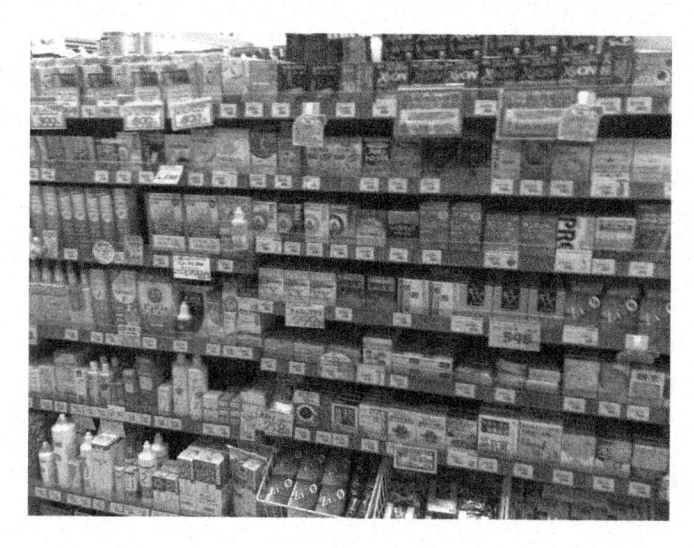

The key to pain pill safety is to do it right. That means carefully checking labels and dosage instructions and understanding the potentials risks and side effects. Many drugs can be habit-forming, causing another issue that I don't have time to tell you about in this book. (Think Prince, Elvis, and other well-known entertainers.) Over-the-counter drugs like acetaminophen, the active ingredient in Tylenol; NSAIDs (ibuprofen, naproxen); and even topical analgesics (capsaicin, menthol, etc.) all have risks and considerations. You must use these with caution, just as you would prescription drugs.

Take Aspirin, for example. It has been available for more than a century. Aspirin is another NSAID, designed to block chemicals in the body that trigger pain and inflammation. It's also used as a powerful anti-clotting agent in the prevention of heart attacks and strokes. But taking too much also makes it more likely to cause issues like gastrointestinal bleeding. So even this 100-year-old drug should be approached with caution.

Prescription drugs such as opioids (hydrocodone, morphine, oxycodone, and muscle relaxers like baclofen and cyclobenzaprine) all work to help relieve pain, but must not be abused. For example, don't take opioid painkillers for longer than necessary for acute pain because large doses can cause nausea, vomiting, and constipation. They can become addictive, and sadly, can even lead to depression, weight gain, extreme fatigue, and even suicide.

As much as we want release from all types of pain, we need to be proactive in getting the best information on what pills we consume. Seek a qualified doctor, read the labels, don't mix or combine certain drugs. When we are in pain, we need to seek the most effective treatment. We need to educate ourselves!

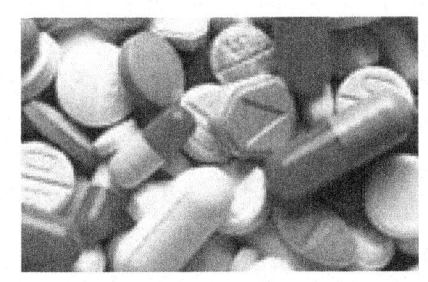

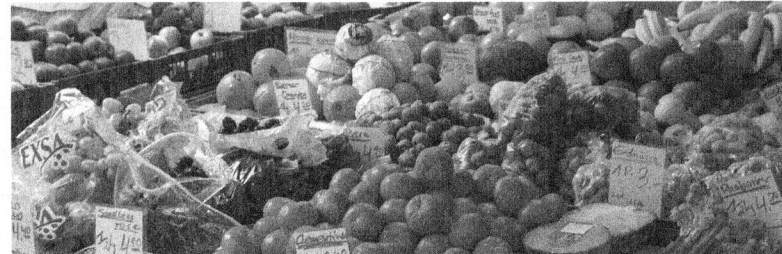

Which type would you try first??

When should we consider taking a dietary supplement or vitamin? The truth of the matter is that, for general health and fitness, a diet that's varied, rich in fruits, vegetables, and whole grains, limits meat to the lean variety, and that's consumed in moderation, provides us with optimal nutrition, and doesn't call for supplements of any kind. But some clinical conditions and special populations (e.g., people with cancer or renal problems, and elderly patients) may benefit from dietary supplementation because of their inability to eat, lack of motivation to eat, or difficulty moderating nutrients because of their disease. In these situations, it is best to refer that person to a licensed/registered dietitian.

Things to remember when you use supplements and vitamins are:

1. Just because a product works for one person doesn't mean it works for everyone, including you.

2. Many people who sell supplements do not have the educational training and credentials in nutrition and dietetics to understand what they are selling you. They are usually commissioned salespeople working for a company.

3. Be critical and curious, and do your homework around supplements and vitamins. Research them on the internet, including their manufacturer claims, and approval by the Food and Drug Administration (FDA), etc.

4. Many herbal medications should not be combined with prescription medications. Always check with your pharmacist or primary doctor.

FINANCIAL GOALS

Another important habit that we should be thinking about is our financial goals. How are you going to stay strong and healthy when you have to stress all the time about having an adequate income when you reach retirement age? There are a thousand books on this topic alone. No wonder. It's an important subject and one for which we sometimes fail to plan.

You wouldn't dream of running a marathon without undergoing months of training. Or betting your life savings on a business venture you hadn't thoroughly researched. When I was researching for this book, I almost did not include any mention of this subject. Then I realized how important it is to save and prepare for our long lives.

In the many articles and books on finances, statistics say that more than half of workers older than fifty-five haven't developed a plan for paying themselves in retirement. Some are entering retirement unprepared.

Let me encourage you to save, because planning late is better than never planning at all. If you are still working, try to save as much as five to ten percent of your monthly income for your future. Start paying off your debts (credit cards, loans, and other expenses). Additionally, start identifying fixed expenses, such as food, housing, insurance, taxes, clothing, family health issues, etc., so you can be more prepared for other big costs, such as new roofs, medical bills, veterinary bills, and automobile upgrades. Keep a budget of everything that goes out of, and comes into, your financial world.

If your company offers a 401(k) plan, take advantage of it. This is a great way to save without too much worry, because you will have more than you had, had you not put into it at all. And that's true if you start an IRA or Roth account, also. If you need to work longer so you have more savings, do it. Then when you do leave work, you will have your savings, Social Security, Medicare, and, hopefully, a great portfolio.

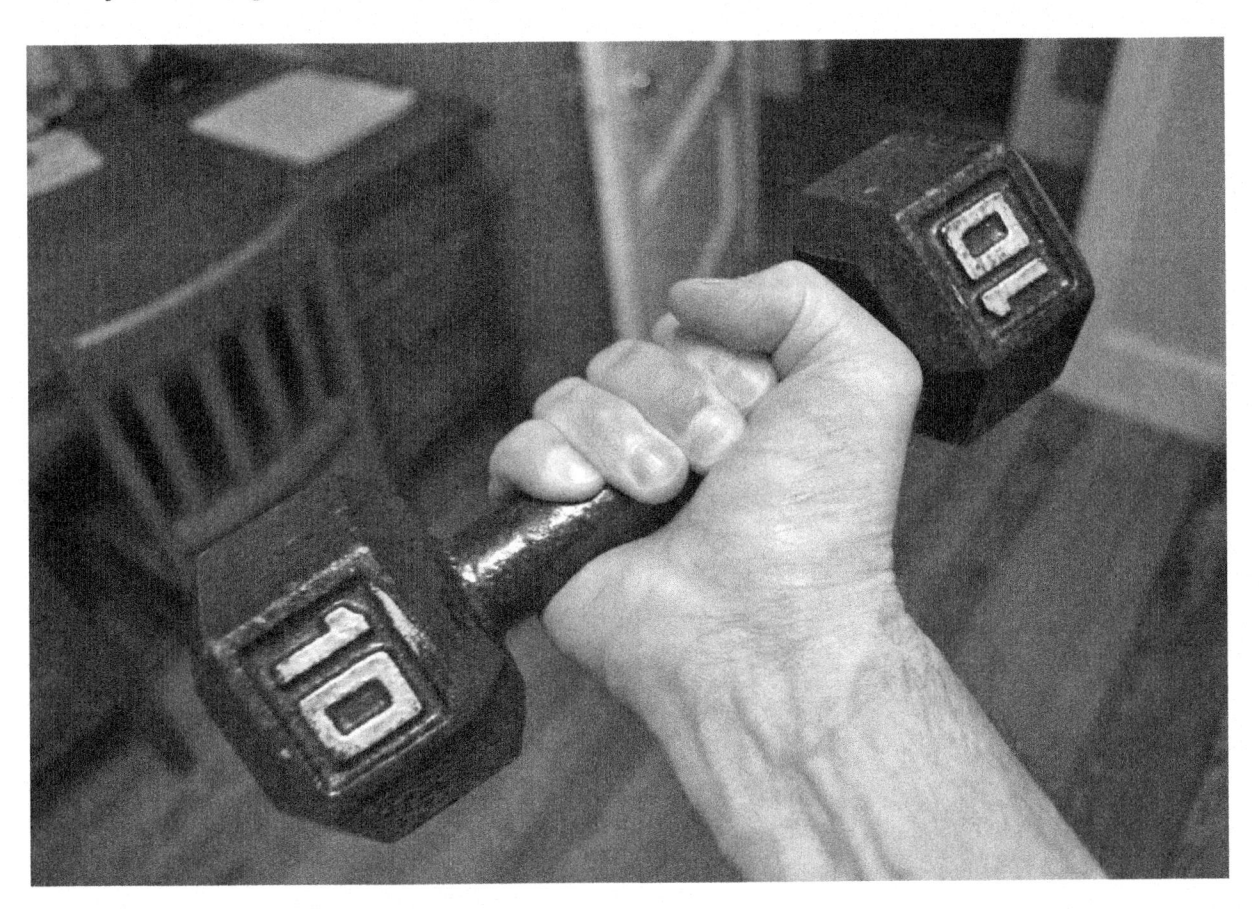

Try to save a tenth of your income

CHAPTER 3:
Exercise and What It Really Takes

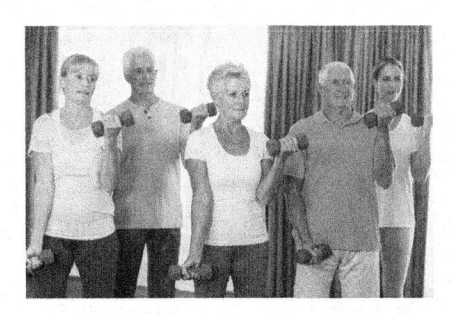

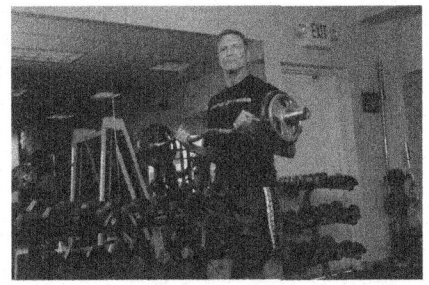

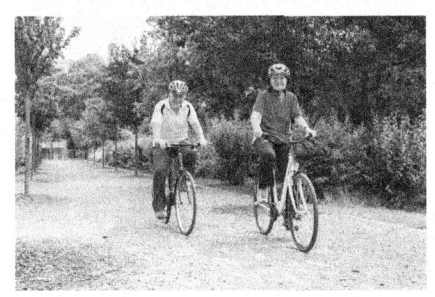

"It takes more than you think!"

EXERCISE: Exercise works to boost vigor, increase longevity, and reduce the risk of dementia, heart disease, stroke, certain cancers, obesity, and other health-related issues. Exercise has even been shown to reverse the symptoms of many conditions and diseases such as coronary artery plaque buildup near the heart and in the blood vessels. Exercise works at a cellular level to trigger healthy changes in every cell type, tissue, and organ system. This can slow or even reverse some of the root causes of aging mentioned above.

HOW BLOOD PRESSURE WORKS IN OUR BODIES: With each beat of our heart, nutrient- and oxygen-rich blood surges from our heart's main pumping chamber (the left ventricle) into an intricate network of blood vessels. These vessels deliver the nutrients and fresh oxygen to our body's tissues and organs. They also pick up carbon dioxide and other waste products produced by our cells. The waste products are removed from our blood by the kidneys.

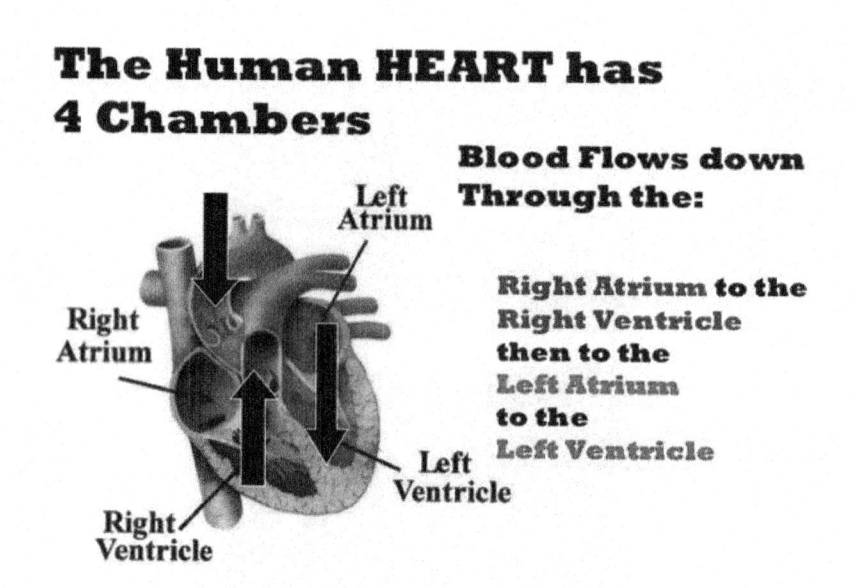

The Human HEART has 4 Chambers

Blood Flows down Through the:

Right Atrium to the
Right Ventricle
then to the
Left Atrium
to the
Left Ventricle

The oxygen-depleted blood returns to our heart and is routed to our lungs, where it releases the carbon dioxide and picks up a new supply of oxygen. The freshly oxygenated and filtered blood is sent back to our heart and is ready to resume the journey again.

A certain amount of pressure is required to maintain this circulation. Your blood pressure is the amount of force exerted on your artery walls to keep your blood flowing, much like the pressure inside a garden hose.

Remember: the main force behind your blood pressure is the pumping action of your heart. To accommodate this surge of blood coming from your heart, your arteries are lined with smooth muscles that allow the vessels to expand and contract as blood courses through them. This maintains blood pressure so that critical organs are supplied between heart contractions.

Blood circulation is a group effort. The kidneys removes the waste products and regulate levels of minerals such as sodium. The central nervous system signals your

CHAPTER 3: EXERCISE AND WHAT IT REALLY TAKES

brain when to make adjustments to the heart rate or blood vessel width. And various other chemical processes help monitor and adjust blood pressure.

Complications come when this complex system doesn't work as it should. For example, the harder your heart muscle has to work to pump blood, the greater the force exerted on your arteries and the higher your blood pressure will rise. When increased pressure continues on a persistent basis, your doctor may diagnose you as having high blood pressure.

Let me also mention that having high blood pressure—or hypertension—gets more common as we age. I will briefly help you understand what this means and what puts you at risk of this condition. Often, there's no identifiable single cause of high blood pressure, but it tends to increase with people who are overweight, and inactive, and also with people with kidney or adrenal gland problems, obstructive sleep apnea, or some kind of congenital blood vessel defects. When high blood pressure is detected in people struggling with diabetes or obesity issues, and/or with those who use tobacco or drink too much, there is a way to manage it.

Treatment of high blood pressure is usually a combination of lifestyle changes and a heart-healthy diet. Continue reading to see what is possible.

A SIDE NOTE FOR FIRST-TIME EXERCISERS: If you have **never** graced the inside of a gym, athletic facility or worked out, you are not alone. Most seniors have never worked out in a gym. They usually did hard, physical work, ate well, and did more walking than we do today. Now they are still alive, and have the chance to live a long life into their eighties, nineties and even hundreds.

So what do you do if you are in this group? Start small, and go big. Assess your current health. **Check with your doctor before starting any fitness program.** And re-read Chapter 1 about the risk categories and proper evaluations you might need before you start. If you want to begin exercising but don't want to belong to a gym, start walking. Ten-thousand walking steps is about a full hour-and-a-half of exercise. Get some good walking shoes, vary your route, walk with a friend, or take a walk with a pet. Walking quickly and as comfortably as you can through a park, along a city street, or in a mall can be just as good as going to a gym. **But you have to do it every day.**

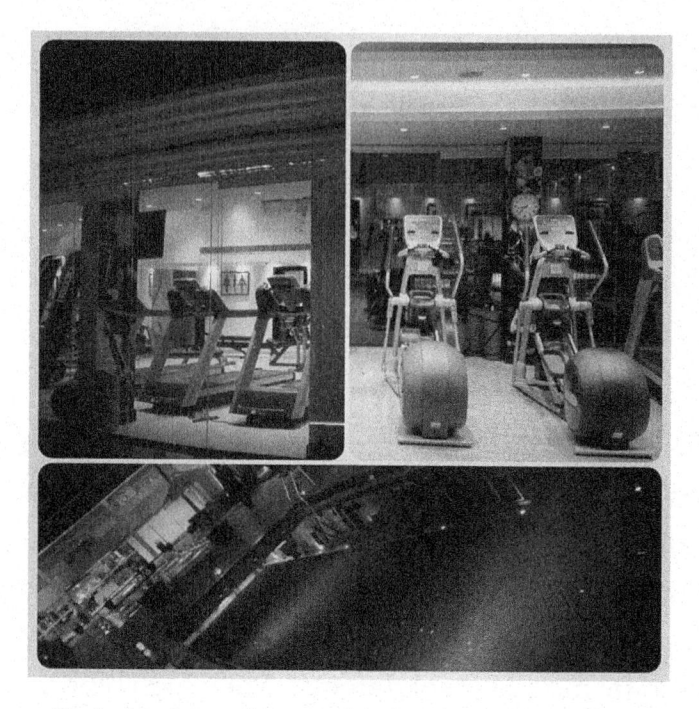

Pick the best fitness facility you can afford

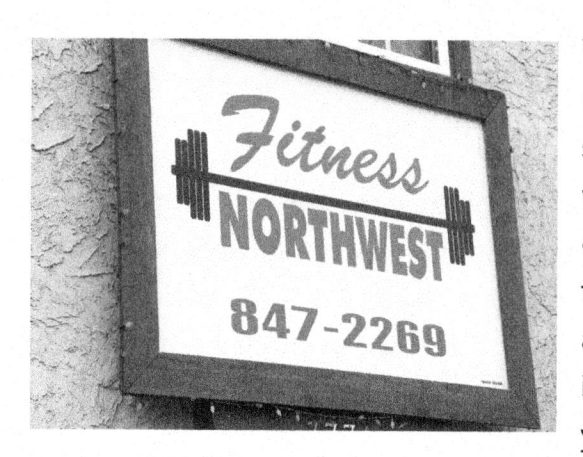

Working out at a gym or athletic facility is much better because you can actually take some days off and still get the workout you want. You learn a lot from these facilities. An example is how to use weights (resistance training) to build muscle and prevent muscle atrophy. Also, you meet like-minded people in classes such as active senior aerobics, yoga, Pilates, aquatics, SilverSneakers@, tai chi, "Bones & Balance," and many more. Finally, the gym option makes you more committed to continue to work out because of the cost and time you put into joining such a place.

I recommend you become a member at a gym near you. Check out the different options and athletic facilities and select one that you think would be a good fit. Your health is very valuable and most gyms are reasonably priced. If you want to swim, choose a gym that has a pool. If you like tennis or handball, choose a gym that offers those attractions. Go online to check out hours of operation and what other items they provide (such as towels, saunas, types of workout equipment, and other amenities). Are they senior friendly? Lots of things to think about, but very important.

CHAPTER 3: EXERCISE AND WHAT IT REALLY TAKES

Did you know that most American adults don't even get the recommended **minimum** amount of aerobic exercise? This is the equivalent of thirty minutes of moderate exercise, such as brisk walking, or fifteen minutes of vigorous exercises such as jogging or swimming, five days a week, plus two sessions of strength-training to build muscle. That's the minimum.

TIPS FOR SUCCESSFUL GYM WORKOUTS:

What we should be getting is a **maximum** of sixty minutes of moderate to vigorous exercise five days per week that includes at least three days of strength-training. To age healthfully, add more strength-training, stretching, and balancing to your program. Also, add that new habit of change that I've been talking about. Go for the benefit of exercise. Here are **five tips to boost your success—so you can reap the benefits of exercise:**

1. Lift weights. Strength-training is critical for older adults to help prevent age-related bone and muscle loss. In fact, if time is limited, shorten your aerobic activity to make time for lifting weights.

2. Don't overdo it, at first. Exhaustion or extreme soreness will make exercise seem like a punishment, not the rewarding experience it should be. When you first work with weights, start on the right path by having a qualified trainer show you the correct way to move weights for the best results. Incorrect use of weights can cause injuries, especially for beginners. Keep it simple, not complicated.

3. Set goals. Be specific about what type of exercise you're going to do, for how long, and how often. An example of this might be: I'm going to lose fifteen pounds in six weeks by working on compound weights three to four days a week for thirty minutes each time and by including aerobic workouts the other thirty minutes for a total sixty-minute workout. Aim for improvements and reward yourself for success.

4. Enlist support: Round up exercise partners (a spouse, family member, or good friend) and/or join a club where you can express your objectives and share your improvements with like-minded people. Explain your goals to family and friends so they can provide encouragement. Make it social!

5. Make it fun and share your results. If you find your method of regular exercise dull or too complicated, try and make it more interesting by working out with people of like-mindedness. Laugh if you make mistakes, and ask questions. If you think you're doing something wrong, ask a trainer or instructor for advice on proper form and movement. Always focus on your goals. Keep challenging yourself with other people who are doing the same thing, and give them praise as much as they give you praise.

Add some type of stretching and balancing exercises after your workout. This is important, because maximizing your post-workout downtime is the surest way to reach any fitness goal. Let me briefly tell you why.

It has to do with recovery, or the process by which your body rebuilds itself. The recovery method you use will reenergize your muscles, and balance your central nervous and hormone systems. It comes in two distinct forms: passive and active.

Passive recovery occurs when your body is at rest. This can include sleep, diet, and applying compression. Active recovery happens when your body is in motion: walking, light lifting, or using a stationary bike after a leg day. Both forms are equally important for optimizing returns on your workout because they target different aspects of muscle regeneration, or repair. Active recovery is the crucial step we skip. If you worked the weights hard or rowed for an hour, you can't just hit the showers, call it a day, and expect your body to magically bounce back to peak form. I recommend a yoga, Pilates, or tai chi class on your off days.

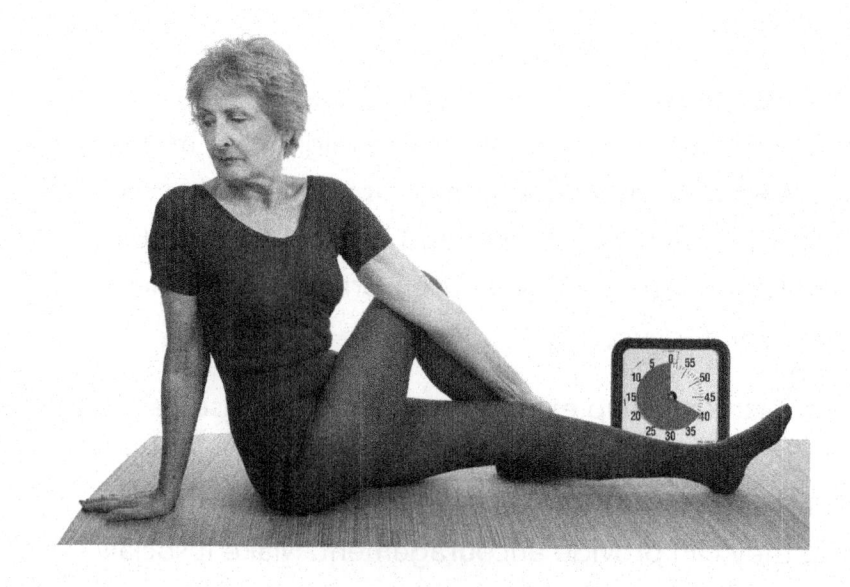

CHAPTER 3: EXERCISE AND WHAT IT REALLY TAKES

Don't be afraid to do workouts on the floor with a thick mat or rug. Getting on the floor or an elevated table for stretches and back exercises are what a physical therapist will sometimes make you do to recover from health issues. Also, ask your instructor for ideas that might work on your stretches. Perhaps a foam roller will help ease the tightness in your legs or back, or a massage will help for overall muscle stress in the chest, arms, shoulders, etc. Take advantage of all that is out there for yourself—you have earned it. And remember that the secret to aging well is exercise. Research has linked exercise to the prevention of some twenty-five health problems.

I also want to mention how you should focus on your exercise. Small improvements to the way you move your body while you exercise are very important. Poor posture or poor gait throws off the spine's natural curves. This can lead to back, knee, and hip pain and injury. It's never too late to change your posture. Try not to slouch when standing or sitting. Follow the habit of relaxing your shoulders, hips, and knees. Tuck in your stomach when you walk. Limit the time you spend sitting or doing things that put stress on your spine. When you work out with weights or are in an aerobics class, a good personal trainer or instructor will notice your posture and gait each time you move. I always look for these things when I instruct a class.

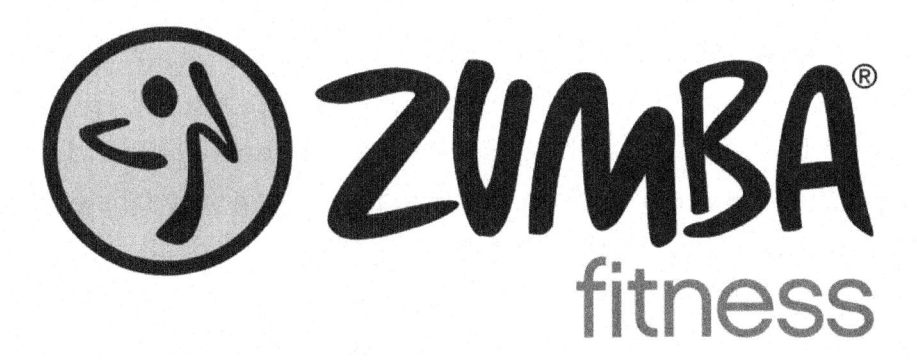

Before I go to nutrition, I would like to give you a little information about the exercise regimen that I do. It features sixty minutes of weight-resistance exercises three days a week, and another three days of cardio. I use weights that challenge me, but not weights that are so extreme that I get injured. If I train with others, I use heavier weights. Safety issues are always to be taken into consideration. For women and older clients who might be working out with weights, there are physiological difference to be considered. Men's bodies and the amount of weight they can sustain are different from women's. Also, if you are just starting out with weights, the amount you use is very important to prevent injuries and help you to come back the next day. Please go slow, be smart about your weights, and always get a doctor's OK before you begin a program. Be smart!

Breathing is another key to a successful workout. Proper breathing during any type of exertion is extremely important. People are often tempted to hold their breath during heavy exertion, which is called the Valsalva maneuver. **Never hold your breath while working out.**

Here's how to do it:

1. Relax your abdominals slightly.

2. Breathe deeply enough that your belly—not your chest—rises and falls as you inhale and exhale.

3. Continue this technique at your own pace to meet your oxygen needs during exercise.

How to **Breathe During Exercise** | SparkPeople
www.sparkpeople.com/resource/fitness_articles.asp?id=1424

If you are new to weight-training, then you will have a lot on your mind: which exercises to use, the location of the equipment, the weights to be used. This can all cause you to have poor breathing issues. Here is the key to understanding the proper time to breathe when working with weights. When you exhale, you are doing the concentric phase of the workout (exertion); when you inhale, you are doing the eccentric phase of the lift (relax). During a bench press, for example, you should exhale as you push the weight up and inhale as you lower it. During bent-over rows, you should exhale as you lift the weight and inhale as you lower it.

Many people tend to breathe from the chest and not the stomach. You can improve your recovery time and fully oxygenate the body if you learn to breathe deeply through your stomach via the diaphragm, which is located at the base of the lungs between the chest and abdominal cavity.

CHAPTER 3: EXERCISE AND WHAT IT REALLY TAKES

Here is an average three-day gym workout that I might do.

Monday: Let's say I'm doing leg exercises. I will warm up enough to feel slightly loose and increase my breathing by spending ten to fifteen minutes walking on a treadmill, or using a stepper or a rowing machine. As we age, we need to warm up more, not less. I sometimes even do all three of these machines for a full range of leg warm-up. Then I will do a complete flexion of the legs, which means I will squat down, flexing at the hips, while keeping the spine in normal alignment, until the thighs are almost parallel to the floor. I will return to the standing position when I go to extension, and that completes the squat. To avoid tearing muscles when practicing the squat, do some stretching exercises by crouching deeply while holding onto a stable support, such at the post of a weight-training machine.

Proper breathing when you squat is important. If I do squats with weights, I will use a Smith Machine for support of the hips and the spine. The Smith Machine is a piece of equipment used in weight-training that consists of a barbell that's fixed within steel rails, allowing only vertical movement. Free-weight squats are better for younger people, but as we age, the Smith Machine really helps. Have an instructor work with you when you first use one.

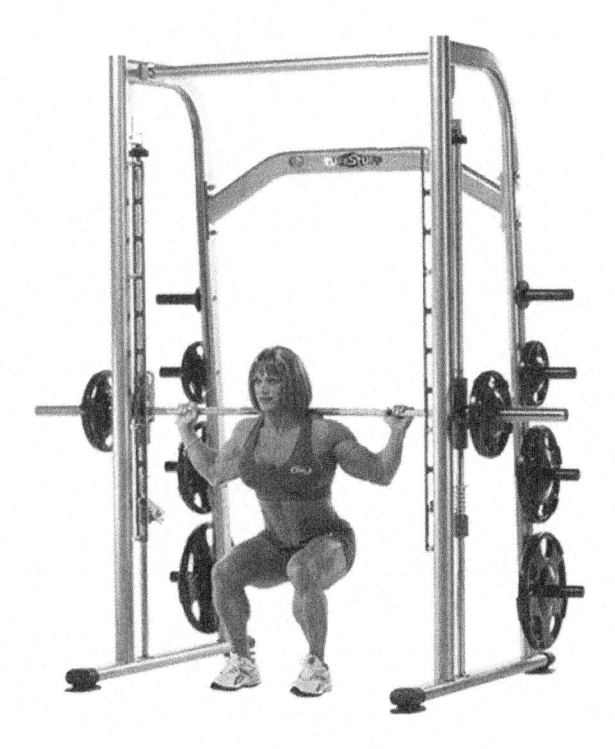

(This is a Smith Machine)

After squats, I may do a leg curl or a leg-extension exercise. A lying, seated, or standing leg-curl machine is perfect to work the back hamstring muscle group and gastrocnemius area. Again, a good personal trainer would be able to help you in this. Using the leg-extension machine is the best exercise for isolating the quadriceps, or the front of the leg muscles. This type of movement is recommended for beginners so that they can develop enough strength to move onto more technically demanding exercises. Machine adductions/abductions, and standing or seated calf raises round out my leg day. I will do three or four sets of twelve to twenty reps for each of these exercises. This is more than what the ACSM requires, but this is my workout.

Wednesday: I might do chest and arms this day. I would warm up with the rowing machine, or a very light lateral or parallel bar dip to open up the anterior deltoid and pectoralis muscles. This also helps me warm up the triceps and forearms. I start with an incline bench press with either a bar or dumbbells. It is your choice which one you want to use, but these types of presses will provide variation contractions that affect the anterior deltoids, the serratus anteriors, and the pectoralis minors differently. Next, I might do a bench press or a dumbbell fly exercise.

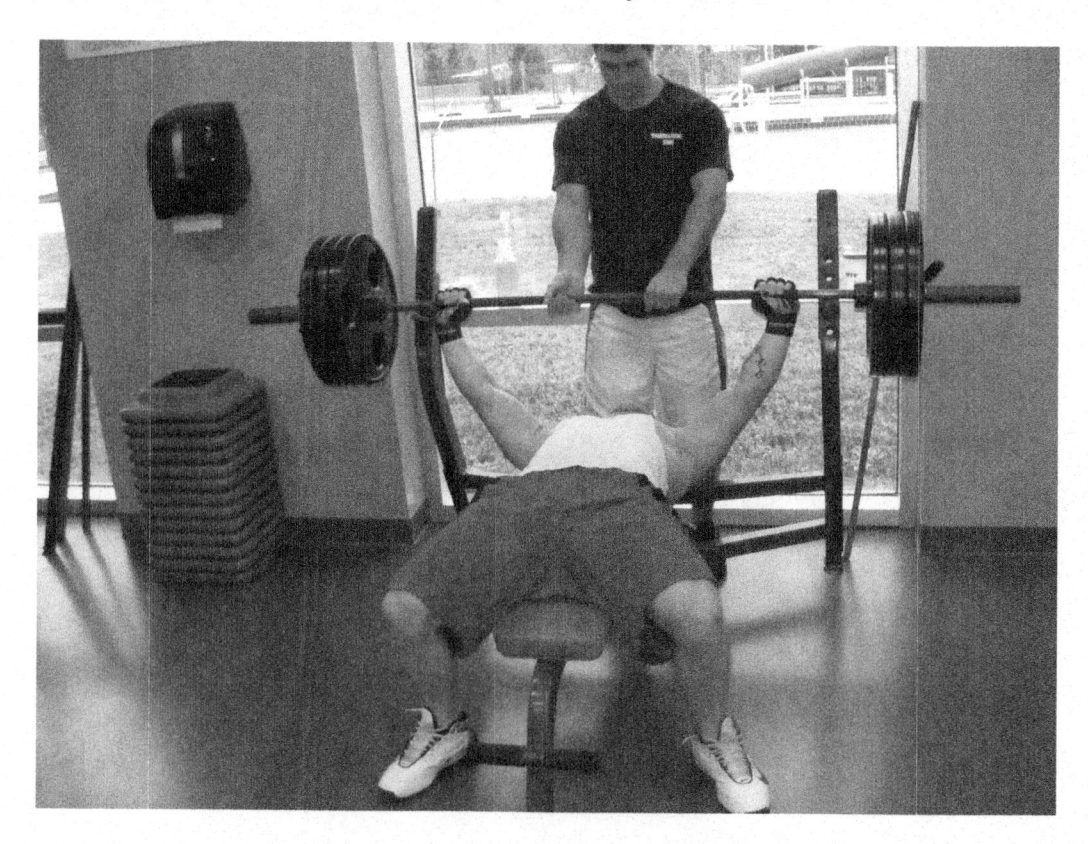

CHAPTER 3: EXERCISE AND WHAT IT REALLY TAKES

Again, check with a trainer for the correct way to do these exercises. To round out my chest workout, I may include a pec deck fly or cable crossover exercise (again, in three or four sets of twelve to fifteen reps with a good amount of weight).

To begin the arm exercises, I start with dumbbell curls or concentration curls. Dumbbell curls can be done like a hammer, with a relaxed hand grip and the palms facing each other. Inhale and raise the forearms together or alternately.

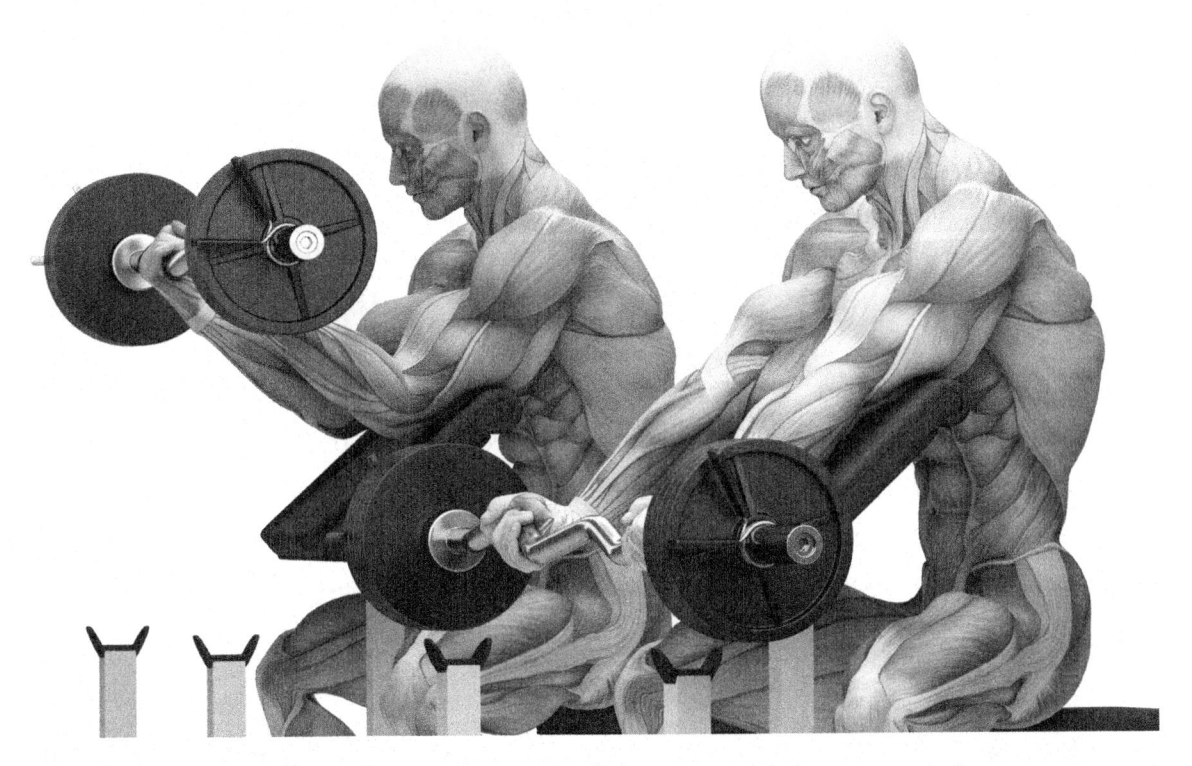

Exhale at the end of the movement.

PLEASE NOTE: When you do any exercise, please watch your breathing.

Another good arm workout is the preacher curl. Sit with the arms resting on a support pad and grasp the bar with an underhand grip. This is one of the best exercises for isolating the biceps. For the triceps, I do a standing push-down cable machine. This method is done by facing the machine and grasping the handle with an overhand grip, keeping the elbows tucked into the body, extending the forearms downward and holding an isometric contraction for one or two seconds. There are other variations to work the triceps, such as lying dumbbell triceps extensions, one- or two-arm overhead dumbbell extensions, triceps kickbacks, and several more. With the arms, I do fewer sets and reps, usually two to three sets and ten to twelve reps with a good amount of weights.

Friday: I will do shoulders/back and abdominal exercises. After warming up for ten to fifteen minutes, I will start with the seated dumbbell press.

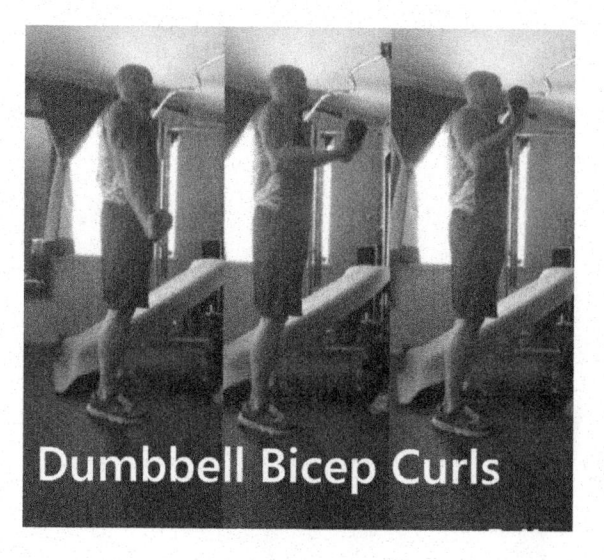

Dumbbell Bicep Curls

This exercise is a good way to work the deltoid area, the trapezius, and serratus anterior muscles. **If you are unfamiliar with the words that I use in this book, please look them up in any anatomy book. This will help you understand areas of the body that may or may not make sense to you.**

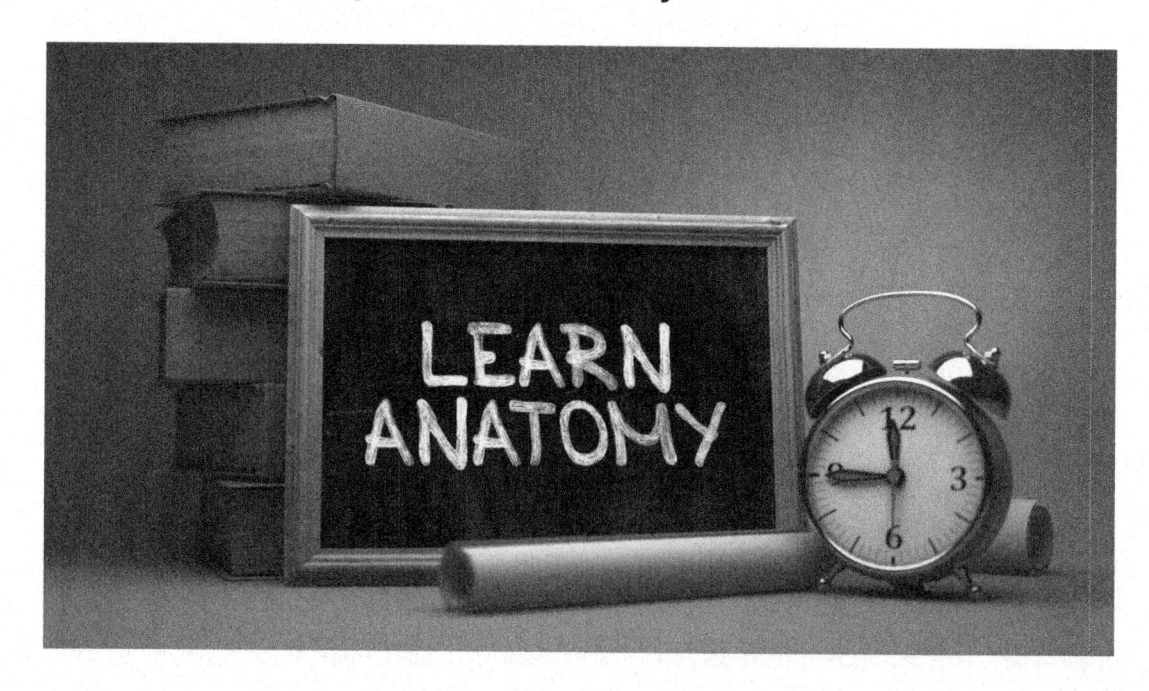

CHAPTER 3: EXERCISE AND WHAT IT REALLY TAKES

Back to my workout. Make sure you have a backrest to prevent you from having an excessive arch in the back. You can also perform this exercise standing, as long as you keep the back straight, thus avoiding excessive curvature of the lumbar spine. Another shoulder exercise are the lateral dumbbell raises. To do this correctly, stand with a straight back, with the legs slightly apart, arms hanging next to the body, and hold a barbell in each hand. Raise the arms to horizontal, with the elbows slightly bent. Use very light weights until you grow stronger. You might alternate this exercise with a front-arm raise, or with a Pec deck rear-delt machine. For part of the back area, you can do barbell or dumbbell shrugs to round out your workout.

For the abdominal exercises, you can start with crunches. I do an oblique exercise that brings my right elbow to my left knee and, alternately, my left elbow to my right knee with each crunch. Another one is the lying reverse abdominal crunch below.

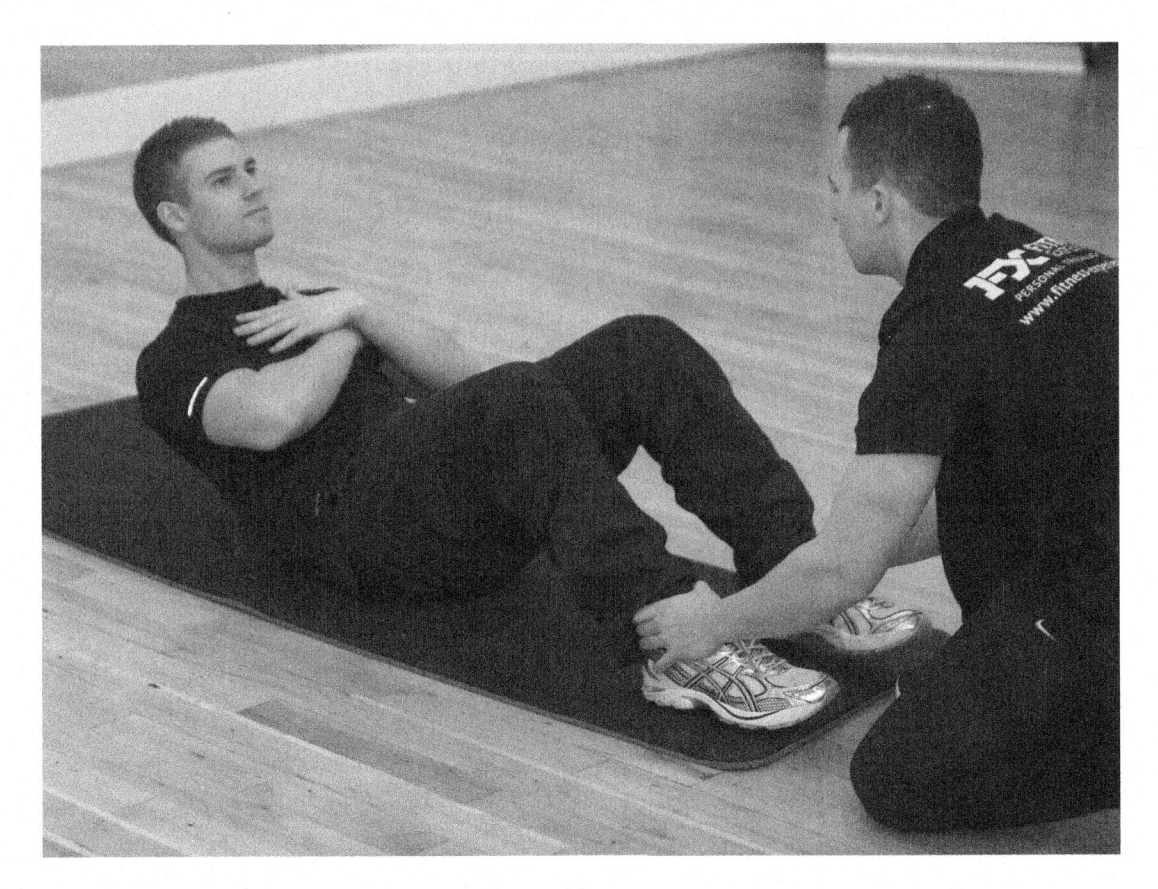

Be careful how you do your abdominals so you get the best benefit. I do ten to fifteen reps with each of these exercises. Planks, bicycle cross-overs, incline leg raises, and other variations for the core are important for a strong back and to prevent a lumbar curve that could force the intervertebral discs forward and cause increased pressure at the posterior lumbar vertebral articulation, which can cause lower-back pain. In other words, the correct position for the abdominals is a rounded, not an arched, back.

I typically do my cardiovascular exercises when I'm teaching my active senior classes. I teach these classes every day, and some are more extreme than others, so I get enough movement. I can get a good workout in with just fifteen minutes of cardio. I may instruct the class with dance steps, aerobic movements, etc. Jumping jacks, running in place, and side-to-side movements are all part of the workouts. Sometimes, I even use weights. I do all classes with music.

When I work at senior living communities, I do not do jumping jacks, running in place, etc., because these kinds of exercises are contraindications to certain individuals' safety and common sense. I end up doing more balance exercises for these communities because their needs are different than others.

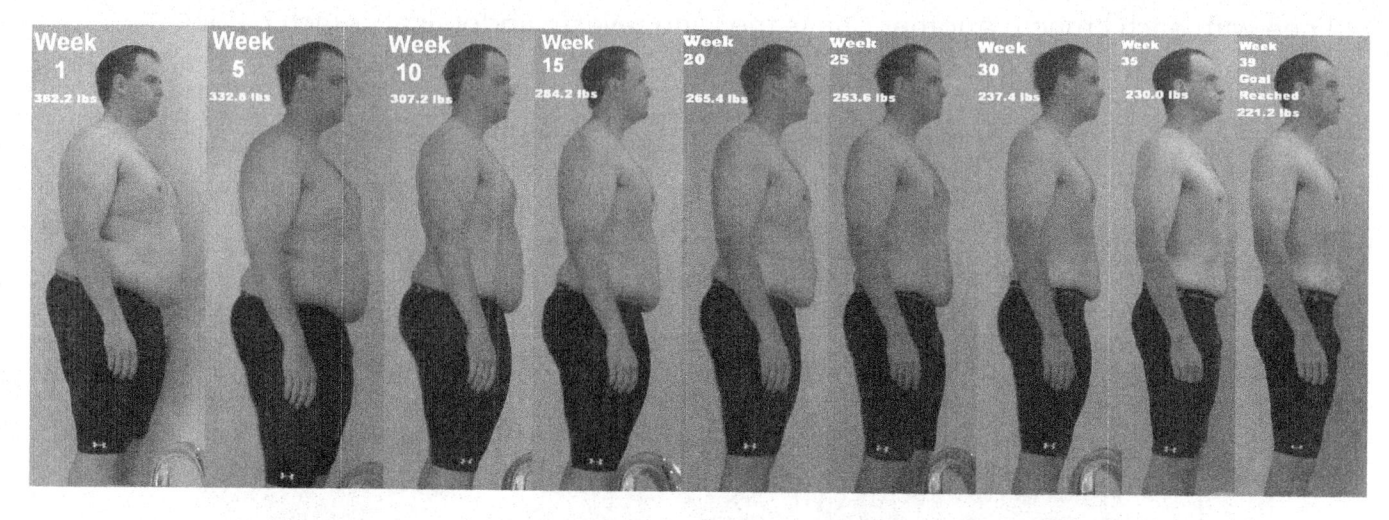

You can see changes in just weeks... even with your posture!

CHAPTER 4:
We Are What We Eat

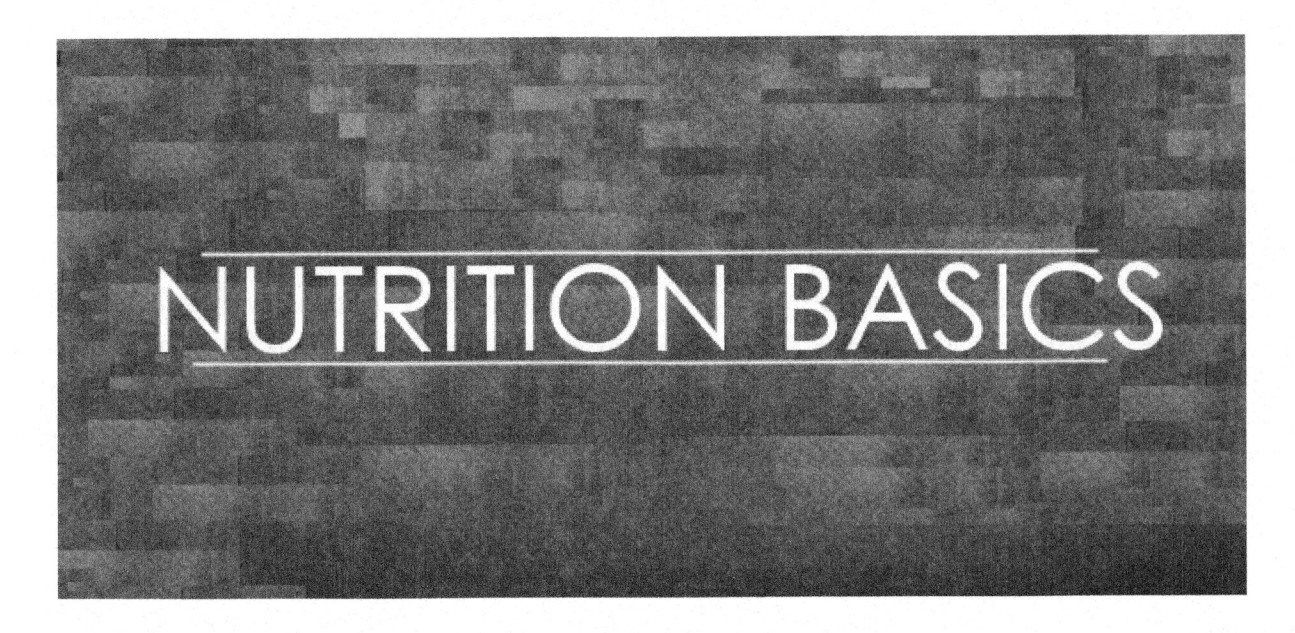

NUTRITION BASICS

NUTRITION: The next focus is your nutrition. You may be wondering why nutrition comes after exercise. It's quite simple. Research has found that what you eat is a big deal regarding what you look like, how you feel, and what energy level you have for exercise.

You have read about how important nutrients are for your overall health. Food is a strong primal part of our lives. It has to be for our survival. Go on line and look up "list of diets" in Wikipedia. You will find hundreds of diets—some that work, and some that are only "fads." I won't mention any of the latter. A desire to lose weight is a common motivation for a person to change their dietary habits, as is a desire to maintain an existing weight. Many weight-loss diets are considered by some to entail varying degrees of health risk, and some are not widely considered to be effective. Eating behavior is the key to understanding your nutritional needs.

Remember: eat foods that are good for you. A diet that is rich in fruits, vegetables, whole grains, fish, and lean meats in moderation can provide you with optimal nutrition. Before we mention more about some of those foods that are good for you, please break the bad habits that ruin your diet. The old joke about being on a "see-food-diet" (i.e., whenever you see food, you eat it) harbors more than a grain of truth. The pleasure and satisfaction you experience when eating delicious food becomes linked in the brain with the sight and smell of that food. When you encounter those sights and smells again, it activates a powerful neurological pathway deep within the brain. You might not decide ahead of time to eat those French fries and that cheeseburger, but the sight of them—even a picture on a menu—taps into a deep well of stored associations. The aromas, flavors, and fun you had while eating them formed a conscious instinct in your mind that you've *got* to have them.

You may not have known this about calories, but if you consume 3,500 calories a day, you gain one pound. Let's say you go to a nice restaurant and order a six-ounce steak? That's 450 calories. Next to the steak are some potatoes with gravy and veggies: another 500 calories. Then you order an eight-oz beer or wine. Another 450 more calories. Also at the table is some bread and butter, salt and pepper, and a condiment for the steak. Chalk up another 600 calories. So far, you have consumed a total of 2,000 calories. Then you have another beer (wine) and some dessert, maybe a nice piece of cake with ice cream. That's a total of 850 more calories. So it's not quite 3,500 calories, but you have gained almost a pound in one sitting. If you include your breakfast and lunch food, you probably ate more than 3,500 calories in one day.

The trouble with diets and counting calories is that most of us soon backslide and wind up regaining what we lost—and then some. That's why some researchers relate all our troubles to the brain. What they're finding is that diets fail because they set people up to battle their own biology. You can't control your genes, but you can control the environment—or, more specifically, the place where you buy and consume your foods. When you go to a restaurant, the sights, smells, and atmosphere can overwhelm even the best intentions. You end up eating and drinking more than you had planned. We have a strong primal urge to overeat.

On top of all this is junk food from other sources, such as convenience stores, vending machines, and grocery stores. Our resources to purchase food are many: from the local mom-and-pop shops to the huge warehouse stores like Costco, Winco, and Walmart. Farmers' markets are a good place to shop, but even there we end up exercising that primal urge to buy discretionary foods like cookies, cakes and candies that are nothing but empty calories. A University of Illinois study found that we squander more than fifty percent of our monthly food bills on empty calories, just because we purchase the first things we see.

Here are three ways to shop smarter and thriftier so you can increase the nutritional power of your purchases at supermarkets:

1. Always shop with a list, and leave the junk foods and empty calories off it so you're not tempted.

2. Look around the stores and stick to the outside aisles where fresh fruits, vegetables, and the leanest cuts of protein foods are displayed.

3. Read the labels on prepared foods. When you do, you start to see what most of them contain. Eliminate those foods that have added sugar, syrup, or non-100-percent whole grain in the first five ingredients.

Every time you pass by brownies in the grocery store or the candy jar at work, you have to override your instincts, and at some point your resistance is apt to falter. Here's how to make this easier for you.

Re-think will power. New brain science tells us that diet advice based on willpower alone might be doomed for failure. Experts now believe that food cues create such a strong primal urge in our subconscious and that the best defense is to **avoid them entirely**. Avoid the brownies, fries, cheeseburgers, and center aisles in grocery stores. Toss the junk foods from your pantry, fridge, and any other places you store your food. "**Out of sight, out of mind!**" This is the only behavior that can help the brain help the body recover from unhealthy eating.

Now, having said this, let me give you peace of mind. Your goal is to monitor your eating level, not to go completely overboard. **You can have a cheat meal from time to time.** This helps avoid the stress of dieting. We can't completely override the desires we have in our brains and completely stop eating the sweets and snacks we love, but which may not be so healthy for us.

The next problem we have is not just *what* we eat but *when* and *how often*. The research linking weight and meal frequency is fuzzy. A bodybuilder should probably eat more often and consume slightly more foods that are based on proteins like lean poultry, fish, and meats, but cut back on breads (or starches) and dairy, and add maybe more vegetables, than someone who is focused only on diet and not the growth of their muscles. Studies suggest that it's not the number of meals you eat that matters, but the total number of calories you consume. It's important that these foods include proteins, complex carbohydrates, and healthy fats. If you're watching your waistline, eating three to five meals a day with a healthy snack thrown in will curb hunger pangs. This is about 400 to 500 calories per meal. So if you eat five small meals a day at 500 calories per, that's 2,500 calories, not 3,500 calories, which is a pound. If you eat fewer calories, you will begin to lose weight. Does this make sense to you?

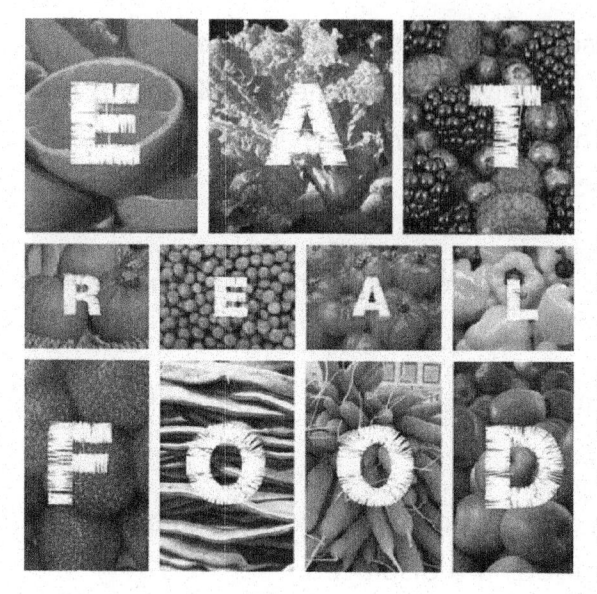

Stick with those foods that are nutrient-dense, and that are a "rainbow" of different-colored produce. Think blues/purples, like blueberries and blackberries; reds, like tomatoes and watermelon; oranges/yellows, like carrots and cantaloupe; greens, like kale and spinach; browns, like potatoes and nuts; and whites, like garlic and cauliflower. Nature provided these rainbow colors, and it's no coincidence that most white vegetables have been known to support heart health, or that orange and yellow produce helps make your immune system bulletproof. Some other color foods help clear cancer-causing toxins from the body; others create oxidants that boost brain health; and others improve circulation.

Always eat breakfast. I have protein, carbs, and healthy fats in the morning. Hard-boiled eggs (without the yolk, sometimes); steel-cut oats with some cinnamon, blueberries, cherries, or other healthy fruit; some nuts; fresh-cut red/yellow peppers; and a cup of coffee and water are my main diet in the morning. Notice there are no breads, butter/jam, bacon, fried eggs, milk, or other cereals, like I used to eat before I turned 50. I eat these, but in moderation and on my cheat days. I also take multivitamins and other supplements (when I remember, which is most days).

CHAPTER 4: WE ARE WHAT WE EAT

Don't skip meals, and drink enough water throughout the day. As we get older, dehydration is a big concern. Remember, we are nearly seventy-five percent water, so we must always keep ourselves hydrated, especially in the morning when we get up. You can drink coffee or tea, but it's much better to replenish the body with water, first thing. Fatigue and irritability can stem from dehydration. So DRINK YOUR WATER!!!

Lunch is the next step that should contain protein, carbs, and fats. I usually have some lean chicken or fish, veggies, and some fruit. The chicken or fish is usually baked. I don't eat much beef, so it's my choice that my main diet is fish or chicken (about three or four ounces). I try to balance my protein with whey powder, and will add blueberries or a banana sometimes with this drink. I'll eat a CLIF bar, maybe some tart cherries, or an apple, or cut-up peppers, with another hard-boiled egg if my time for lunch is rushed and I have a need to eat something. Eggs are not on everyone's diet list, but I'll have a little egg white (the protein in the egg) to keep my sugar level under control. I prepare my foods a couple of days ahead, so it's easy for me to grab them before going to my classes.

I typically eat dinner before six o'clock. I can snack later if I feel hungry before going to bed. My dinner is fish or chicken together with steamed veggies such as onions, cabbage, broccoli, and fresh colored peppers. Notice the rainbow colors? I don't eat much more than this. For a snack later on, I'll have air-popped popcorn, rice cakes with avocado or peanut butter spread, or just an apple. Sometimes, I make a special protein bar that has carrots, blueberries, walnuts, nutmeg, allspice, cinnamon, salt, egg whites, whey protein, oat or almond flour, baking soda, and water for a tasty snack. That is usually all I need to maintain my weight and muscle mass.

Another thing to mention is that the meat and dairy industries have deceived the public into believing people need a lot of protein. Re-read the last few pages, because I do mention protein, but you can avoid eating animal products if you're vegan by including legumes, avocados, nuts, and other B-12 vitamins with folic acid products. Include those rainbow-colored foods, too.

If you're not able to eat good nutritional foods every day, you may want to add multivitamins, omega-3s, or supplemental pills to help you—but, there is no magic pill that you should rely on. The best way to stave off the inevitable is with good habits, such as eating a healthy, balanced diet and exercising regularly.

There's so much that could be written into this book about nutrition, exercise, anti-aging supplements, health tips, etc., but the motivation to follow all of them is still up to you.

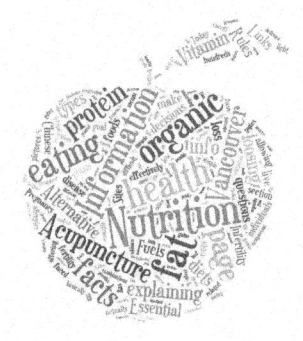

I could show you thousands of exercise pictures, give you hundreds of pieces of advice about nutrition, health, and fitness, but it's still up to you to follow your pledge to see them through. Remember, you should exercise at least three to five days a week, sixty minutes or more each time. You should do at least three days of strength-training and two to three days of cardio. You should be watching everything you put into your mouth. You should be eating balanced meals each day and all in moderation and according to what your goals are. To lose weight, cut back on the calories and portions you consume. To build strength and muscle, increase your protein and watch how much fat and how many carbs you consume. For each goal or habit you focus on, you need to be smart and determined to succeed.

Overall, a balanced diet cuts your risk for diabetes, obesity, some cancers, and other problem diseases such as Alzheimer's, dementia and Parkinson's. Eat plant-type foods often and fill up on healthful veggies, beans, and protein. Adding fruit for dessert can help slash your chances of getting these diseases. In fact, researches from Harvard, the Cleveland Clinic Wellness Institute, and even the Global Alzheimer's Association Interactive Network are all preaching the same. These plant-based foods attack the tissue in hormones and feeds the cells that absorb blood sugar. This helps get elevated glucose levels under control. The final step is exercise!

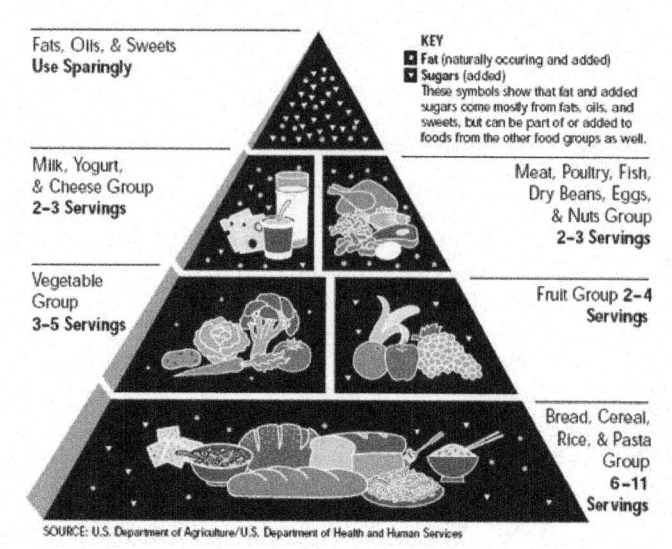

Working your muscles with weight-resistance training will help lower elevated blood-sugar levels. Working your muscles encourages them to pull blood sugar from your bloodstream, even if muscle cells are insulin-resistant. It also makes those cells more sensitive to insulin, so they grab more blood sugar. That's why I stay healthy. I exercise with weights.

CHAPTER 5:
Focus Also on The Brain

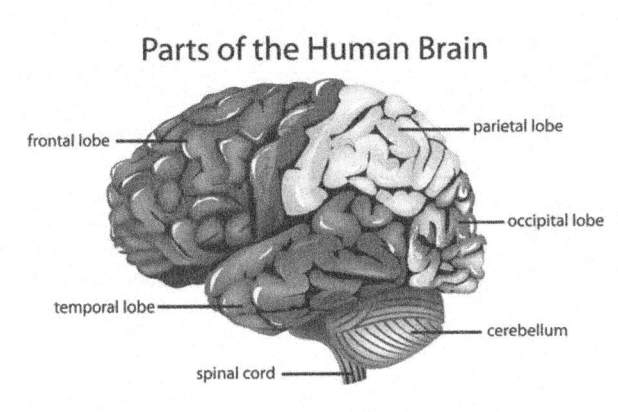

Another exercise to focus on is your brain. Yeah! The muscle in your head needs as much training and exercise as your lower body. Doing crosswords, playing cards, building puzzles, playing board games, and engaging in other brain teasers is critical to keep you young and focused. Playing a musical instrument, reading, math games like Sudoko, video games, and, if you have to watch TV, game shows such as Jeopardy and Wheel of Fortune will help you keep your mind active and young. Let me explain.

A growing body of research has proven that people who play games become more empathetic, helpful, and sharing toward others. They learn more quickly, develop greater mental focus, become more spatially aware, estimate more accurately, and multitask more effectively. Think of all the times you've played something with someone. You probably enjoyed the thrill of victory or defeat. Either way, it's another habit that helps you reach the fifties and beyond clear headed and focused. Even exercise classes with others of like-minded level and ability also works the mind because you challenge yourself with your peers. When you explain to the new members how the exercise works, you learn their names. You try to improve and hopefully encourage them to improve. It's pure empathetic inspired help and it's all good!

You can impact your brain function and cognitive abilities by making simple tweaks to your daily routine here and there. The first, of course, is to exercise.

Exercise encourages our brain to "work at its optimum capacity" and to release proteins and other chemicals that promote and benefit our cognitive functions and learning. By improving blood flow and oxygen to the brain, you make it work faster and more efficiently.

Sleep is another essential need for your brain. It enhances your memory and helps improve your performance of challenging skills. It "resets" your brain to look at problems from a different perspective and can impact your ability to think clearly more often. You need at least seven hours of sleep most nights. Even a mid-day nap now and then has been found to boost and restore brainpower.

Watch what you eat, because approximately sixty percent of our brain is composed of fats. The omega-3 fat docosahexaenoic acid (DHA) is an essential component of our diet. We need it because our bodies can't produce it, so we must get it from our daily intake of foods. It's found in seafood, eggs, nuts, and liver. Other fats come from avocados, coconut oil, and vitamin B12. To deprive our brain of these types of fats will cause it to starve because it won't have the glucose-converted energy it needs to function normally.

Another big help for the brain is to listen to music and challenge your mind and body, one of the simplest methods of boosting your brainpower. Listening to music while exercising can boost cognitive skills and improve mental focus among healthy adults. Most exercise classes are conducted with music in the background. My classes always include a metronome rhythm and variety of music. The music's motion, regular succession of tempo and movement, and rate of speed are great boosters to exercise.

So protect your brain! Protect your mental health, just as you would your home and personal values, or your life from danger. As I work with many types of people to help them live longer, I can only say that we must always focus on our health. We may lower our risk for diseases like dementia and Alzheimer's—problems that are on the rise as we age. All that I have written above can be put into **5 simple brain-health reminders that can prevent these risks. They are:**

1. Eat healthily, because the right foods help boost mental energy and improve concentration. Eat more fish, especially coldwater fish filled with the omega-3 fatty acids that are important to brain health.

2. Exercise. A number of studies suggest that exercise is a good way to protect your brain. Exercise pumps our brain with fresh blood and oxygen and decreases inflammation in the hypothalamus, something that can cause problems as we age. A sedentary lifestyle makes us more prone to cognitive decline.

3. Break bad habits like smoking, excessive drinking, and even mixing interactive medications because they've all been linked to mental decline and other side effects.

4. Watch your stress and get enough sleep. Developing relaxation techniques such as deep-breathing exercises, meditation, and letting your body rest (sleep) for at least seven hours each day will have a significant effect on your memory. Yoga, tai chi, massage, and Pilates are also excellent stress releasers.

5. This one is so important: **Be a socially active person.** When you are socially active, you're more mentally alert and you're doing things that challenge your mind. Your ability to remember names, locations, dates, and all those people and things with which you come into contact on a daily basis will keep your memory strong.

Remember, the first fifty years are the lifestyle habit years. How you managed those years will help or hinder your next fifty years. Your habits make all the difference. If you've done well with your health—by instituting practices of good eating; exercise; social, educational, and financial habits—congratulations! Your conquest to reach your goals has been fulfilled! You should live a long life.

But if you didn't do so well with those good lifestyle habits yet, you can see that it's still possible to get them. You can do even better than you have been doing. This small book is for you. Re-read it to focus on your weak points.

CHAPTER 6:
Focus On What You Are Able to Do

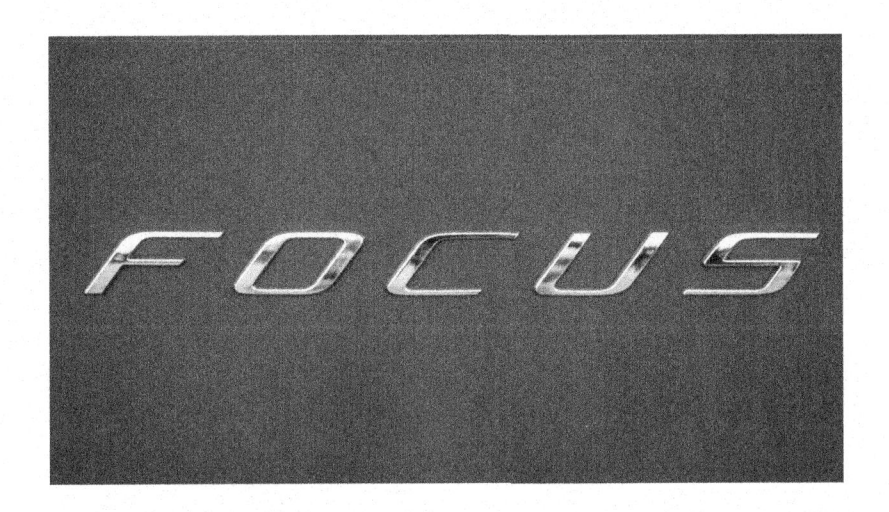

One of the things I do for myself is to focus on what I need to do almost every day for my overall health, especially working out. *Daily Exercise for Overall Health* is an eighteen-point massage I do for myself with no weights. It can be done in about five to ten minutes while getting ready for work, or before bed at night. Do these five to ten reps on each body part.

Daily Exercise for Overall Health

1. **Click your teeth together (move your jaw up and down).**
2. **Use your fingers to apply pressure around your eyes.**
3. **Use your fingers to massage around your face.**
4. **Comb your hair with your fingers (from front to back).**
5. **Massage the upper and lower parts of your ears.**
6. **Reach behind your neck with two fingers of both hands and massage.**
7. **Massage downward along your throat with both hands.**

8. With one hand, reach across the opposite shoulder and bring that hand down your arm to the finger tips. Turn your hand over and move back up to the shoulder. Repeat the process on the other side.

9. Make small circles with your fingers, around your ribs.

10. Focus your fingers on your ribs, stomach, and abs, with big, circular motions.

11. Use your knuckles on the back near your kidneys.

12. Circle in both directions below the belly button.

13. Start with the front hips and press hands downward to the ankles and feet, reverse the procedure on the backside starting at the ankles back to the butt.

14. With your fingers, massage the soles of your feet with small circles.

15. Do relaxed bounces.

16. Take in many deep breaths and swing your arms from side to side.

17. Stand and do cross reaches across the body with knees up, much like cross crunches if you are lying down.

18. Finish with eye circles (with your fingers following your eyes in both directions).

If you try this eighteen-point daily massage exercise for your body and review the three points and the five strategies listed below, you should reach the level of health that only the few obtain.

Focus on these three points:

1. As far as your diet goes, remember to cut back on your fats and carbs and watch your calories and portions. Start eating healthily. Balance is the key. Up your intake of rainbow-colored foods for even better results.

2. If it's exercise that's your focus, increase your level of physical activity. Ask for help from a certified trainer or instructor. Remember to do at least sixty

minutes of exercise five days a week. Do at least two to three days of weight-bearing exercises with two to three days of moderate to extensive cardio. Remember to do two to three sets of eight to twelve reps for best results when lifting weights. Always check with your doctor when starting a new program.

3. If bad habits like smoking, drinking, using recreational drugs, or taking too many pain pills, etc., are your focus, remember that these addictions can be overcome. All things take time, but new habits can be cultivated, with help and counseling. You have the next fifty years to make it happen.

I want you to enjoy your life like I enjoy mine. Have fun working on your goals, and achieving and maintaining GOOD HEALTH.

To help you plan for your long life and to stay independent in older age on your own terms, I will summarize again the strategies that you will need. Remember: being capable of various basic functions such as caring for your daily needs, making personal decisions, managing your finances, engaging in meaningful activities, and keeping your doors of communications and relationships open, are all part of these strategies and goals. Focus on what you're able to do with these goals.

Strategy number 1: Stay physically fit as long as you can. Physical activity is strongly linked to healthy aging and remaining independent. Regular exercise, like I mention in this book, boosts physical health and supports the ability to perform those every-day activities that are essential for independence, such as climbing stairs, gardening, shopping, and carrying objects. It also improves cognitive functioning and keeps you mentally sharp. And it helps prevent falls. Regular workouts help older adults maintain balance and flexibility, build strong muscles, and increase bone density, reducing the likelihood of broken bones, fractures and other physical injuries.

Strategy number 2: Make your health a priority. As we age, any health crisis can lead to a loss of independence. Protect your health. Avoid all those destructive practices mentioned earlier in this book. Find ways to relieve stress. Have regular checkups for your skin and teeth, and manage already established medical conditions. Have your vision and hearing tested more often. All these things are for your health and success in staying independent, **and they must become your priority.**

Strategy number 3: Emphasize healthy eating. Poor nutritional habits are strongly linked to cognitive decline, frailty (showing signs of weight loss, low grip strength, slow walking speed, low physical activity, and exhaustion), and other physical problems that might interfere with independence. Be sure to eat the rainbow style of foods mentioned in Chapter 4. Aim for a nourishing, low-calorie diet that includes plenty of vitamin-rich fruits and vegetables, nuts, and healthy fats such as olive oil, fish, whole grains, and legumes.

Strategy number 4: Stay engaged with supportive social relationships. I see many engaged seniors helping their friends, family members, and others. It goes well with good mental health and mental acuity in older age. There are many ways to enjoy a fulfilling social life. For example, volunteering to help others can lead to greater life satisfaction. Engaging in activities with friends and family in such activities as a shared meal, attending a concert, or playing games can provide for stimulating social interaction. Going to church or temple, or having some other form of spiritual relationship with this beautiful earth is something we all need. Stay engaged!

Doing things for yourself is also important. Learning a new hobby, doing crosswords or Sudoko, or visiting a play or museum may also offer mental stimulation. Staying in touch with others by telephone, e-mail, Facebook, and Skype, as well as through face-to-face encounters, is another way to help counteract feelings of isolation.

Strategy number 5: Remaining independent requires us to be realistic and flexible in all we do. Our financial portfolio can help us extend our independence even more, as unexpected issues come up. This means honestly assessing what we can and cannot do, and getting help when we need it. An example is when we need assistance accomplishing difficult tasks in our home. We need to take a positive approach, and adopt a resilient attitude toward change. If we need to move from our home to a retirement community, a positive attitude is fundamental to self-sufficiency. Remember to consider your quality of life, and if you find you're becoming house-bound and can no longer go out and participate in activities, do things like yardwork, cleaning, and simple maintenance. You might find that your life would be improved in a more supportive environment. You still have your independence, but you don't have to worry about all the other "stuff" that makes life difficult.

"To be or not to be, that is the question."
Do you remember who said this?

REFERENCES:

Aerobics and Fitness Association of America, AFAA Standards and Guidelines for Senior Fitness, All rights reserved, Copyright 2014.

American College of Sports Medicine. *ACSM's Health/Fitness Facility Standards and Guidelines*. 4th ed. Champaign (IL): Human Kinetics; 2016.

Center for Disease Control and Prevention. *Prevalence of Self-Reported Obesity Among U.S. Adults*. Atlanta (GA): Centers for Disease Control and Prevention; 2014.

Cardiovascular health in middle age and beyond: a gift from your genes or is it earned by a healthy lifestyle and within your control? Sci News; 2014.

Phillips SM. Dietary protein requirements and adaptive advantages in athletes. *Br J Nutr.* 2012: 108 (Suppl 2): S158-67.

Life Extension: *The ULTIMATE Source for New Health and Medical Findings from Around The World.* Volumes 17, 18, 19/ Numbers 9, 10, 11; 2014.

Wilmore, Jack H., Costill, David L., and Kenney, Larry W. 4th ed. *Physiology of Sport and Exercise.* Human Kinetics; 2014.

Consumer Reports on Health, Volume 26 Number 2, February 2014, pg. 4-5.

Mind, Mood & Memory, Massachusetts General Hospital, Volume 12, Number 1, January 2016

Mayo Clinic Health Letter, Volume 34, Number 10, High Blood Pressure, pg.1-3. October 2016

All pictures from free clip arts and registered stock only